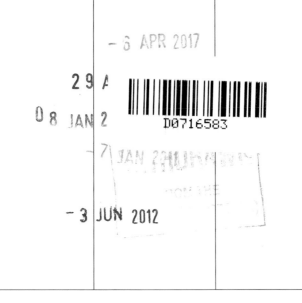

Other titles in this series:

Thorsons Natural Health

Diverticulitis

ARTHUR WHITE
N.D., D.O.

Thorsons
An Imprint of HarperCollins*Publishers*

Thorsons
An Imprint of HarperCollins*Publishers*
77–85 Fulham Palace Road,
Hammersmith, London W6 8JB

First published by Thorsons 1988
This edition published 1997

10

© Thorsons Publishing Group 1988, 1997

Arthur White asserts the moral right
to be identified as the author of this work

A catalogue record for this book
is available from the British Library

ISBN 0 7225 1549 9

Printed and bound in Great Britain by
Caledonian International Book Manufacturing Ltd, Glasgow

Contents

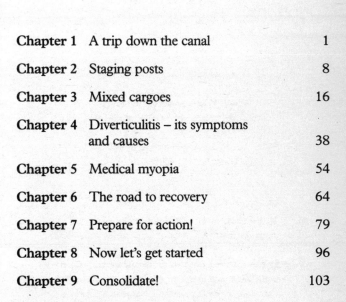

1

A trip down the canal

Although diverticulitis is a condition which afflicts the colon or large intestine, it is a mistake to concentrate attention solely on this small area of the alimentary canal and attempt to treat the bowel lesions in isolation from the rest of the digestive system.

It is just such a short-sighted approach which, as shall be explained more fully in a later chapter, has been largely responsible for the disappointing results achieved by much of the orthodox treat-ment over the years. By contrast, the naturopathic approach sees diverticulitis, along with several other common gastric disorders, as being the end-result of a chain of events which have progressively weakened the various parts of the digestive system until a point is reached at which the weakest link in its complex chain of components finally breaks down under the strain.

Whether the eventual disease crisis is centred in the throat, the stomach, the duodenum, the small intestine, the appendix, the colon or the rectum will depend on many variables, including the patient's age and previous health history and the nature and duration of the predisposing factors. On these also will depend the nature and severity of the ultimate affliction, for example, stricture of the throat, gastric or duodenal ulceration, appendicitis, colitis, diverticulitis, haemorrhoids, or even cancer.

A prerequisite to understanding the nature and causes of diverticular disease and the logic of the naturopathic treatment measures which need to be adopted if lasting relief is to be achieved, is that the reader should have a working knowledge of the complex organs and systems which comprise the digestive tract. To this end we propose to conduct the reader on a guided tour down the alimentary canal.

The alimentary canal

It may surprise many people to know that from the moment food is taken into the mouth to the time when the unwanted residues are excreted from the rectum a distance of no less than 9 m (30 ft) is traversed, a journey that takes between 36 and 48 hours.

The figure on page 4 shows how nature has contrived to package such a complex collection of mechanisms into the confines of the human torso and the various stages at which other vital organs such as the pancreas and liver become involved in the chemical processes of digestion and assimilation.

Entry into the canal is via the mouth where the combined actions of the tongue and teeth break down and partially liquefy solid food so that it can pass easily into the oesophagus (gullet) which, after traversing the chest cavity, enters the abdomen via an opening in the muscular diaphragm which forms the floor of the thorax.

At this point the macerated food enters the stomach where it remains for a period varying from 3 to 6 hours during which time it is churned around by continuous, slow, wave-like contractions of the muscular walls. During this process the food mass is mixed thoroughly with digestive juices secreted by glands in the membranes which line the stomach and further reduced to a porridge-like consistency. Once this stage of the digestive process has been completed the pyloric valve at the lower end of the stomach opens and the pulped food – known as chyme – moves on into the duodenum which constitutes the first 30 cm (12 inches) of the small intestine.

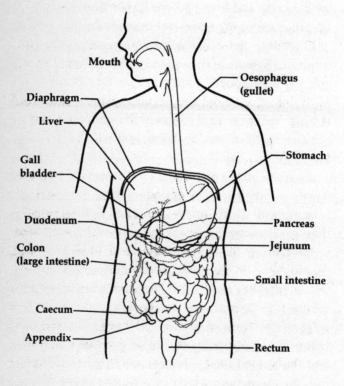

Figure 1 Diagram of the Alimentary Canal.

At this point in the journey a small tributary enters the alimentary canal bringing bile from the liver, via the gall-bladder, and digestive juices from the pancreas. The functions of these complex chemical substances, which will be explained in a subsequent chapter, are supplemented by further secretions from glands in the lining of the intestine itself and by beneficial bacteria which are normal inhabitants of the healthy intestine.

The food, which at this stage is totally liquefied and known as chyle, now begins the longest stage of its journey through the closely packed coils of the small intestine, traversing a distance of some 600 to 700 cm (22 ft) and being propelled by a series of wave-like contractions, a process which is termed peristalsis.

Although in simple terms the small intestine is basically a lengthy, convoluted tube measuring 50 mm (2 inches) in diameter at its upper end and tapering gradually to 25 mm (1 inch) at its junction with the colon, there is nothing simple about its functions. It is at this stage of the food processing conveyor-belt that miracles of chemistry are performed in order to extract nutrients from the chyle, sort them into their various categories and pass them into the bloodstream so they can be conveyed to the tissues where they are most needed for purposes of maintenance, growth or repair. At the same time, any unwanted or potentially harmful substances are rejected and neutralized and then moved on into the large bowel or colon. Entry from the small intestine into the colon is guarded by a valve which opens to permit the passage of waste material and then closes automatically to prevent any reflux.

At its junction with the small intestine, low down on the right-hand side of the abdomen, the colon forms a bulbous pouch – the caecum – from the base of which protrudes a narrow tubular appendage, popularly and appropriately known as the appendix. Until well into the middle of the twentieth century the appendix was often removed by scalpel-happy surgeons. Fortunately, the operation has now gone out of fashion, largely because of a belated recognition by the orthodox medical profession that the removal of an inflamed appendix can sometimes lead to more health problems; the operation does not address the dietetic and other factors responsible for the inflammation in the first place. (This is another subject to which we shall return in a later chapter.)

Continuing our metaphorical journey along the alimentary canal, we have now reached the ascending loop of the colon, which is a much shorter but bulkier tube than the small intestine, having a diameter of approximately 10 cm (4 inches) and a total length of only 1.3 m (4½ ft). From the caecum in the lower abdomen it ascends more or less vertically for some 15 cm (6 inches) before flexing to the left and looping across for a further 50 cm (20 inches) passing just beneath the lower margin of the liver and pancreas. It then descends down the left flank and curves sharply inward to the centre of the pelvis, a further distance of some 65 cm (26 inches) before looping downward to form the rectum which itself measures approximately 12 cm (8¾ inches).

The alimentary canal terminates at the anus where two rings of muscular tissue – the internal and external sphincters – form an effective seal which can be relaxed voluntarily to permit defaecation.

What we have described during this brief exploration of the digestive tract are only the physical components of a remarkable system of organs which, when they are functioning normally, accomplish feats of metabolism and assimilation which could not be duplicated by even the most skilful chemist in a laboratory equipped with the most advanced scientific apparatus.

In the next chapter, therefore, we shall outline some of the extraordinarily complex functions which are carried on, day and night throughout our lives but of which we are totally unaware unless, through thoughtlessness or ignorance, we misuse or abuse our digestive organs to such an extent that they are no longer able to operate efficiently.

2
Staging posts

As was indicated in the previous chapter, the primary function of the alimentary canal is to transport raw materials to a series of staging posts throughout the body where they are processed and utilized according to physiological needs and to collect surplus and waste materials and carry them away for disposal.

In order that we may understand the true nature of the physical defects which characterize diverticulitis and the factors which, often over a period of many years, have caused them to develop, it is necessary to have a working knowledge of the specialized functions of the various organs which are served by the alimentary canal and the complex chemical and physical processes which they are required to carry out in order to keep our bodies functioning efficiently.

The first stage

Although the first stage of digestion takes place in the mouth, the processing plant is in fact triggered into action even before the first mouthful of food is taken.

The 'early-warning system' is set off by the sight and smell of food as a result of which groups of glands situated beneath the tongue and around the throat release a copious secretion of saliva. The latter is fluid which is made up largely of mucus but which also contains a ferment named ptyalin which is responsible for the first chemical process of digestion, that of converting starchy foods such as cereals, bread, potatoes, etc. into sugary substances which can be readily absorbed and assimilated into the bloodstream.

To facilitate this and subsequent phases of digestion it is essential that all food is masticated thoroughly, so that it is ground down and mixed with saliva. Mucus from the latter lubricates and partially liquefies the food and forms it into a small ball which can then pass easily through the throat. During this process a flap of cartilaginous tissue closes over the passage through which air passes from the nose to the lungs to prevent food or liquid from 'going down the wrong way' and causing coughing or choking.

There are important lessons which need to be learned concerning this first salivary stage of the digestive process:

1   Unless food is adequately masticated, i.e. if it is eaten hurriedly and gulped down, it will not be sufficiently softened and lubricated and so will tend to 'stick in the throat'.
2   Similarly, bolted food will not be properly permeated by the ptyalin in the saliva and so the transformation of starchy food into sugar will be impaired.
3   These digestive derelictions will be compounded if they are perpetrated in the course of consuming a very large, mixed meal washed down with tea, coffee, wine or beer.

When the salivary stage of digestion has been completed the food enters the gullet, a muscular tube some 50 cm (20 inches) in length, the walls of which begin to contract and relax to produce peristaltic waves, propelling the food down into the stomach. The fact that the act of swallowing is controlled by peristalisis and *not* by the force of gravity explains why it is possible, though not advisable, for foods to be ingested even by someone who is standing on his or her head!

The role of the stomach

The arrival of food at the entrance to the stomach triggers off a reflex action which causes a muscular sphincter to open and, as the food enters, the walls of the stomach commence a series of slow churning movements. Normally, the regurgitation of food is prevented by the closure of the sphincter. If, however, the stomach lining is irritated by tainted or over-rich food, or by an excess of alcohol or any other potentially harmful substance, a nerve-centre in the brain is alerted which causes the sphincter to reopen and the contents of the stomach will be ejected by a violent and uncontrollable contraction of the diaphragm and abdominal muscles.

The sight and smell of food which activated the salivary glands will also have a similar effect on many millions of glands in the stomach wall which respond by exuding a copious flow of gastric juices. These consist of a complex mixture of ferments and acids which are slowly churned into the food mass and which break down the protein constituents of the meal and prevent putrefaction from taking place in the alimentary canal. These processes may continue for several hours, by which time the nutrients in the semi-liquefied food (chyme) will have been rendered completely soluble.

So far no nutritional material has been removed, for the role of the stomach in the digestive process is merely to churn the food around slowly and ensure that every particle is broken down and mixed thoroughly with the digestive juices. Once this has been achieved the pyloric valve at the lower end of the stomach opens and the slow, wave-like contractions of its walls force the chyme, a little at a time, into the duodenum.

Before we proceed, however, it is necessary to underline further lessons which the sufferer from diverticulitis, or any other digestive ailment for that matter, needs to learn if the nature and causes of his or her problems are to be understood and put into context with the natural treatment measures which need to be implemented if lasting health is to be restored.

Firstly, the digestion of starchy foods which is begun during the process of mastication is normally continued for from 20 to 30 minutes after they enter the stomach, during which time the ptyalin is neutralized by the acids in the digestive juices. Therefore, as we have already explained, if the first salivary stage of digestion is curtailed as a result of skimped mastication or overeating, the gastric acids will more readily check the action of ptyalin, the starches will not be fully converted into assimilable sugars and the nutritive value of the food will be appreciably reduced.

By the same token, a very bulky meal will distend the stomach beyond its normal capacity of approximately 1¼ litres (2¼ pints), thus preventing the muscular walls from functioning efficiently and mixing the gastric juices into the chyme. The all-too-familiar pangs of indigestion are likely to be the least serious consequences because, here again, the whole chain of digestive processes will be slowed down and subsequent absorption and assimilation will be impaired.

Add to all this the dilution of the gastric juices which results from the large quantities of tea, coffee, alcohol, etc. which all too frequently accompany such a meal and it is not difficult to appreciate the tremendous handicap which is imposed on the digestive system as a result of such thoughtless feeding habits. This brief homily is intended merely to prepare the way for a more detailed consideration of the dietetic causes of diverticular disease in a later chapter.

The intestines

Meanwhile, it is time to rejoin the conducted tour at the point where the chyme is being released from the stomach into the duodenum. It is at this juncture that a small tributary, called the common bile duct, enters the intestine, bringing bile from the gall-bladder, which is fed by the liver, and another digestive juice from the pancreas (see figure on page 4). The former consists mainly of a mixture of pigments and salts which play an important part in the digestion of fatty substances, but it also contains metabolic waste products removed from the bloodstream by the liver. The pancreatic juice is an even more complex chemical substance which contains four very potent ferments which respectively (a) break down fats, (b) curdle milk, (c) complete the digestion of starch and (d) continue the task of protein digestion which was commenced in the stomach.

All of these crucial functions are further supplemented by secretions from millions of tiny, hair-like projections, called villi, which cover the inner walls of the intestine giving it a velvety appearance, Despite their minute size – they are barely visible to the naked eye – the villi are incredibly complex structures. Each one, in addition to containing tiny blood-vessels, muscle tissue and secretory glands, is capable of absorbing nutrients from the food material, now completely liquefied as chyle, passing along the intestine.

The peristaltic contractions which began in the gullet and continue to propel the semi-liquid chyme through the stomach and into the duodenum are now carried on by the muscular walls of the small intestine. These propel the liquid chyle towards the next and final staging post – the colon or large intestine which it enters via a valve situated in the wall of the caecum. As the processes of digestion and assimilation have been completed, the surface tissue of the colon differs from that of the small intestine by being less convoluted and devoid of villi. Its primary function is to extract much of the water from the chyle and transfer it to the circulatory system via a network of blood vessels in the walls of the colon, leaving a semi-solid residue of waste material to be moved slowly towards the rectum for excretion via the anus. To facilitate this final stage of the digestive process the lining of the colon is covered by a layer of mucous membrane, the profuse secretions from which act as an effective lubricant.

Before moving on, however, there is one further and crucial facet of the digestive process which needs to be mentioned, namely, the part played by beneficial bacteria which, in healthy individuals, inhabit both the small intestine and the colon. In the former they produce ferments which help to complete the digestion of carbohydrates and in the latter they break down protein residues and prepare them for excretion. Their health-promoting functions do not end there, however, for they also have the valuable capacity to manufacture some of the components of the vitamin B complex. We shall have more to say concerning these bacterial benefactors later on.

It is necessary, now, to turn our attention to the raw materials which we feed into our bodies. This will help us towards a clear understanding of the nature of food and the complex functions which it is required to perform in order to maintain the delicate metabolic balance upon which bodily health depends. Such a preliminary appreciation of the basic principles of human nutrition is essential if the reader is to recognize the logic of the self-treatment measures advocated here and apply them confidently and conscientiously.

3

Mixed cargoes

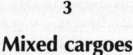

Throughout the 70 years or so which constitute what is generally regarded as being the normal human life-span, the tissues of our bodies are subjected to a continuous process of break-down and renewal. It needs little thought to appreciate that the materials needed for the maintenance and growth of our bones, muscles, skin, nerves, blood and other specialized components which make up the human body can only be derived from the raw materials provided in the form of the food we eat, the fluids we drink and the air we breathe.

Apart from Man and the animals which he has domesticated, all living creatures are guided by natural instinct in the selection of nutrient materials. Anyone who has even a passing experience of caring for animals will know that it is virtually impossible to persuade them to eat foods to which they are not accustomed and which are not approved when subjected to the critical senses of sight, smell and taste.

Intelligent Man, however, has long since neutralized these natural censors and the natural foods which, only a few generations ago, constituted the basic diet of the majority of people have in the meantime been manipulated and 'de-natured' to such an extent by commercial processing that much of what is now consumed derives more from the chemical laboratory than it does from the soil. Moreover, the air we breathe is heavily polluted by gaseous industrial emissions and exhaust fumes, and even the water we drink has to be subjected to a variety of chemical processes before it can be considered fit for human consumption.

Since the health and functional efficiency of the human body depends so largely on the nutritional qualities of the food we eat, if we are to repair the damage which has been inflicted on the colon and caused diverticular disease it is important to look first at the basic materials needed for the rebuilding process.

Thanks largely to the widespread preoccupation with the problems of obesity, much public attention has been drawn by the press to the potentially harmful effects of nutritional imbalance. Radio and television programmes frequently stress the fact that an excessive consumption of fats, sugar, salt, etc. may be at least a contributory factor in the incidence of specific diseases such as high blood pressure, diabetes and coronary heart disease.

Laudable as all this may be, it does have one serious drawback – it implants in the public mind the idea that specific dietary excesses are responsible for specific bodily disorders, whereas the overriding principle in human nutrition is that bodily health and functional efficiency are dependent upon a balanced diet containing a wide variety of nutrients in their natural form and combinations. Given such a diet, the raw materials which enter the alimentary canal will, as explained in the previous chapter, be processed at a succession of staging posts and separated into their component parts. These can then be transported, speedily and efficiently, to whichever organ or tissue is in need of them. Any excess may be stored for future use as required, or discarded and eliminated.

Only when the system is grossly overloaded with the commercially de-natured products of the modern food factories is the vital metabolic balance destroyed and the complex functions of the various staging posts thrown into disarray. Burdened with a mass of useless and often harmful substances, and deprived of essential nutrient materials, their complex operations are disorganized and it is inevitable that, sooner or later, the tissues and organs which are in need of maintenance and repair will suffer and break down.

It is a tribute to the remarkable tolerance and adaptability of the human organism that it is able to withstand such abuse and misuse for many years and still continue to function with some degree of efficiency. Even more remarkable, perhaps, is its capacity for repair and self-healing once provided with the right conditions and materials.

What makes a healthy diet?

To understand the nutritional factors which lead to a breakdown in the walls of the colon and cause diverticulae to form, it is essential to start with some idea of what constitutes a healthy diet, including the way in which nutrients maintain and repair the complex tissues and organs on which our health – and indeed our very lives – depend.

To simplify a little a subject that is so complex that even the most expert nutritionists have never been able to unravel all its many mysteries, we will confine ourselves to a brief survey of the basic food components – proteins, carbohydrates, fats, vitamins, fibre and water.

Proteins

When proteins are mentioned, most people's thoughts turn to animal products such as meat, fish and dairy products. Until relatively recently, orthodox nutritionists claimed that these were the only 'first-class' proteins. This led to the widely held belief that meat is an indispensable dietary component and much was made of athletes and body-builders who were reported to consume vast quantities of steak, eggs and other animal derivatives in order to build up their muscles and improve their performances. It is true that the structure of animal tissues is very similar to that of the human body which, so far as our present knowledge is concerned, is composed of 20 amino acids. These are the basic protein building-blocks needed, in various combinations, for the construction and maintenance of muscles, nerves, bones, glands, hair, skin, etc. Of these 20 there are believed to be 8 so called 'essential' amino acids which can only be derived from dietary sources. Provided that an adequate supply of these is obtained from our food the body is able to manufacture for itself the remaining 12 'non-essential' amino acids.

Unlike animal proteins, those derived from vegetable sources, such as nuts, pulses, cereals, yeast, may be deficient in one or more of the 8 essential amino acids and it was this fact which gave rise to the myth that they were nutritionally inferior to animal proteins. It seems that the 'scientific' nutritionists were so preoccupied with their test tubes and bunsen burners that they failed to recognize that a vast proportion of the world's population thrives on a vegetarian diet and that many more have only a very limited access to animal proteins. In physical development and athletic prowess these nutritionally 'under privi-leged' people more than hold their own against those who have unlimited access to 'first-class' animal pro-teins. Once this anomaly was brought to their notice, the scientists had second thoughts and it is now rec-ognized that man does not live on meat alone, and that any amino acid deficiency in one vegetarian food is readily made good by other components of a balanced dietary.

It cannot be stressed too strongly that the keys to healthful feeding are *balance, variety* and *moderation,* and in no other respect are these factors more impor-tant than in regard to the protein content of our meals, and especially in regard to meat and other animal derivatives.

Fats

As a logical extension of this aspect of human nutri-tion we will now turn to the subject of dietary fats, because there is little doubt that an excessive con-sumption of fats of all kinds, and animal fats in par-ticular, is a significant factor in the alarming increase in the incidence of coronary heart disease in the wealthier Western communities.

It is a demonstrable fact that the fat content of foods in their natural state is almost invariably low, which implies that the body's need for this particular nutritional component is equally modest. Dietary imbalance in this respect results from the widespread practice of extraction and concentration on fats and oils and the universal use of the end-products of these processes in the cooking and preparation of our daily food. Virtually the only vegetable foods which have a relatively high fat content are nuts, soya beans, avocado and olives, all of which are eaten rarely, if at all, by most people.

By contrast, the majority of dishes which compromise the conventional Western diet have a very high fat content. For example, many people would no doubt be surprised to learn that fish and chips, perhaps one of the most popular dishes in the UK, has an average fat conent of 10 per cent, while the figure soars much higher for a mutton chop (60 per cent), a pork chop (50 per cent), bacon (50 per cent) and sausage rolls (36 per cent). Perhaps even more surprising is the fact that sweet mixed biscuits have a high fat content (31 per cent), as also have digestive biscuits (20 per cent), milk chocolate (38 per cent), and flaky pastry (42 per cent).

Clearly, any meal which includes foods such as these will have an abnormally high fat content and this will be increased still further if it is followed by a steamed pudding (21 per cent), or Cheddar cheese (34 per cent) with cream crackers (33 per cent) and butter (85 per cent) or margarine (85 per cent).

The metabolic crime which such as excessive fat consumption perpetrates against the liver and arteries in particular is compounded by the fact that most fats in these dishes will be derived from animal sources and so are 'saturated fats' as distinct from most vegetable fats which are 'unsaturated'. It is not possible to discuss in detail here the very complex chemical and physiological implications of these terms. Suffice it to say that most nutritional and medical authorities are now agreed that is is the saturated animal fats – those from meat and dairy produce – which are likely to be most damaging to human health and should therefore be consumed only in the strictest moderation. A simple, rule-of-thumb method of distinguishing between saturated fats and the unsaturated variety is that the latter are usually supplied in liquid form, whereas the former remain solid at ordinary room temperatures. In the context of healthy eating, however, the distinction is academic since the body's normal requirement of this nutrient will usually be met adequately by the fats contained, in the natural proportions and combinations, in the simple wholefoods which constitute a balanced, healthful diet.

Carbohydrates

In terms of human metabolism, fats fall into the same category as carbohydrates since their principal function is to generate heat and energy. This leads us inevitably into a consideration of the very controversial subject of calorie values, a subject which features prominently in the interminable discussions concerning the widespread problem of obesity.

It is because carbohydrates – the starch and sugary foods – have tended to dominate Western diets during the past half-century or so that they have attracted so much unfavourable attention and are so often listed among the 'foods to be avoided' in the slimming régimes which have become a regular feature of the popular press and television programmes.

Certainly, there is ample evidence to confirm the view that a high-calorie diet which contains an excessive proportion of white bread, sweets, cakes, pastries, white rice and pastas, sweetened breakfast cereals and all the other commercially processed products made from white flour and white sugar, has been responsible to a large extent for the high incidence of obesity and such diseases as diabetes, dental caries and coronary heart disease. It is common knowledge that dental decay is rife among children of all ages and there can be little doubt that the development of what is euphemistically termed a 'sweet tooth' begins in the cradle when an irritable baby is passified by being given a bottle of sweetened milk or fruit juice, or even a dummy dipped in syrup, or is fed on an artificial substitute for its mother's milk which consists of refined cereal sweetened with white sugar.

By the time such a child reaches school age he or she will have become accustomed to being given sweets, chocolate, ice-cream and other sugary confections as presents or rewards for any achievements or as an incentive to co-operate with parents. The teeth are the first victims of the resulting sugar addiction and as a consequence there are few if any adults who reach middle age without losing at least half of the 32 'permanent' teeth because of dental caries. What is probably less well known is the fact that 15 per cent of people over 50 years of age are known to be afflicted with diabetes and it is suspected that many more cases exist but are undiagnosed.

It needs to be stressed, however, that it is not the carbohydrate foods as such which are responsible for this state of affairs, but the nutritional deficiencies of the commercially refined starches and sugars which have come to play such a disproportionately high part in human nutrition. Sugar, like fat, occurs in natural foods in limited quantities and in balanced combination with other nutrients, and its chemical constitution can vary significantly according to the nature of the food in which it occurs. Most fresh fruits, for example, contain sugar in the form of fructose in combination with various vitamins, minerals and fibre and diluted by a very high water content – approximately 80 per cent – which of course serves to limit the amount of sugar which can be consumed at any one time from this source. On the other hand, the white sugar which is sold in such vast quantities today is in the form of sucrose and is derived mainly from sugar-beet, having been extracted, concentrated and chemically 'purified'. In their text-book, *Human Nutrition and Dietetics*, Davidson and Passmore describe white sugar as 'one of the purest chemicals regularly produced in large quantities by modern industry; it is practically 100 per cent sucrose and contains no other nutrients such as minerals and vitamins.' They go on to say that 'its very attractiveness is a danger in that it tends to displace other more nutritious foods from the diet.'

In order to illustrate the effects of sugar addiction – for that is what is implied – it needs to be appreciated that until the eighteenth century, sugar even in its raw, unrefined state, was a luxury which only the wealthiest could afford. However, in the last hundred years or so the *average* consumption of sugar in the UK has risen at an extraordinary rate to well over 50 kg (1 cwt) per person per annum! It is not surprising, therefore, that the human metabolic system should have been so seriously disrupted by what, in evolutionary terms, is virtually an overnight revolution in the demands inflicted on its chemical processing organs and that vital tissues and functions should have suffered as a result.

If, however, sugar must be regarded as public enemy No. 1 in regard to human health, it is only marginally more harmful than the refined white flour which is not only consumed in such large quantities in the form of white bread, cakes, pastries, puddings, pies, pastas and sweetened breakfast cereals, but which is also widely used by the food industry to bulk out many of the tinned and packeted 'convenience foods' which fill the shelves of the food stores. Moreover, since our concern here is specifically with the causes of diverticulitis, and indirectly with those of constipation and other bowel and digestive disorders, it has to be conceded that white flour is even more culpable than white sugar. Here, again, we are referring to a product which has only been widely available to the general public since the early years of the nineteenth century. It was then that the industrial use of power and machinery and other technical 'advances' made it possible for the millers to extract the bran and the nutritious germ from the wheat grain during the milling process and sell them as a profitable by-product. From then on the price of white flour fell progressively and white bread replaced the coarser but more nutritious wholemeal varieties as a staple food in nearly all Western communities.

The nutritional effects of this revolution were very considerable. Firstly, the extraction of up to 30 per cent of the wheat-grain meant that virtually all the bran and much of the mineral and vitamin content were removed, thus seriously reducing the nutritional value of the food and disrupting its chemical balance. One of the implications of this process was clearly demonstrated when outbreaks of beri-beri among troops in the First World War were shown to be directly caused by vitamin B deficiency in the white bread which formed a dominant part of their diet. Little was done to remedy the situation until 1942 when the Government ordered the introduction of National Flour with an extraction rate of 85 per cent, compared with the previous standard of 70 per cent. The motive, however, was not to safeguard the health of the consumer but to reduce the weight of grain that was being imported from North America at a time when our merchant shipping was being decimated by enemy submarines. At the end of hostilities, however, the permitted extraction rate was reduced from 85 per cent to 80 per cent, and ten years later, in 1956, an even greater reduction was authorized, restoring the flour to the pre-war low level of 70 per cent extraction.

To their credit, however, the authorities had recognized that the refined flour had significant nutritional deficiencies and the millers were therefore compelled to 'fortify' all low-extraction flour with certain B vitamins, iron and calcium (common chalk). Regrettably, these supplements could be added as pure chemicals, and no consideration was given to the subtle metabolic differences between the synthetic substances and the natural nutrients which had been removed from the wheat or the effects of bleaching agents and other chemicals which are used during the refining processes.

It needs to be stressed, also, that there are almost certainly gaps in our knowledge of the nutritional properties of all staple foods, including wheat, and so there may well be other, as yet unidentified, vitamins and other nutrients which are either depleted or destroyed. The effects of this on human health are as yet unsuspected.

Fortunately, the flour-milling regulations specifically exclude 100 per cent wholewheat flour from the fortification requirements. Consequently any loaf described as 'wholemeal' or 'wholewheat' can be relied upon to contain all the natural wheat-germ, bran, vitamins, minerals and other nutrients and be free from the synthetic substances which are added to all other loaves, whether they are described as 'brown', 'farmhouse', 'wheatgerm', 'fortified', 'granary', or any other ambiguous and often intentionally misleading term.

Before leaving the subject of carbohydrates it is important to reiterate that these foods form an essential part of a balanced, health-promoting diet. It is only when they are commercially de-natured and taken in excessive amounts to the exclusion of other foods that they may constitute a potential health problem. This subject is discussed again later when I describe the dietetic and other therapeutic measures which need to be adopted for the treatment of diverticular disease.

Vitamins

The fact that, as was mentioned previously, a deficiency of some of the B vitamins can cause a serious disease such as beri-beri underlines the vital role of these nutrients for human health. Yet it was not until the early decades of the twentieth century that the existence of these substances was finally confirmed. Prior to that time, discerning nutritionists had demonstrated an undeniable link between inadequate nutrition and certain so-called deficiency diseases. For example, records show that more than four centuries ago it was known that the inclusion of citrus fruit in the diet effectively prevented scurvy, a serious disease which claimed the lives of many sailors, explorers and others who were compelled to live for very long periods on a diet which was often devoid of fresh fruit and vegetables. It was only in 1932, however, that vitamin C was isolated from lemon juice and its chemical structure elucidated.

Similarly, cod-liver oil was used in the treatment of rickets in the mid-nineteenth century, but the responsible nutrient – vitamin D – was not isolated until 1931. Discoveries such as these spurred the nutritional scientists into activity and led to the discovery of many more vitamins, the nature and properties of which have since been confirmed and described at great length in research papers and nutritional text-books.

Unfortunately, however, the reaction in orthodox medical circles had been to concentrate increasingly on what may be termed 'fragmentary nutrition', based on the assumption that a deficiency of a vitamin or other specific nutrient is largely responsible for a certain specific disease or group of symptoms and that the logical treatment is to prescribe large doses of the missing substance. Thus, children suffering from rickets (weak bones) are given massive doses of vitamin D and patients suffering from pernicious anaemia are given iron injections in the form of concentrated liver extract.

In their obsession with research into the minutae of various nutrient properties the food scientists have been blinded to what naturopaths have always maintained is the fundamental principle of healthy dietetics: the body should be provided with all the essential nutrients in their original forms and combinations as they occur in natural foods, and so be allowed to select and utilize those needed for its vital functions and either excrete excesses or store them for future use.

Fibre

The fallacy of attempting to rectify the harmful effects of nutritional deficiencies by supplementing or reinforcing the patient's diet with large doses of extracted and concentrated nutrients is particularly relevant to the sufferer from diverticulitis and other bowel disorders. Until the middle years of the twentieth century the orthodox medical profession was still insisting that such patients should eat only what was termed a 'low-residue diet'. This consisted of white bread, white rice and pasta, cooked and strained vegetables and fruits and milk puddings, in other words, the very foods which are now recognized as being a major cause of these patients' symptoms.

Yet for more than half a century the naturopathic pioneers had maintained that the bran in wholegrain cereals and the fibrous tissues of vegetables and fruits served an essential purpose in stimulating bowel functions and that these foods should be included in the diet of sufferers from constipation and related disorders such as colitis and diverticulitis. When, eventually, the logic of this reasoning was finally accepted by the medical profession it was hailed as a 'scientific breakthrough'! Predictably, the low-residue diet was replaced by the high-fibre diet, but instead of sufferers from bowel disorders being advised simply to eat wholegrain cereals, fruit and vegetables they were told to 'supplement' their fibre-deficient diet with relatively large quantities of bran. A senior surgeon, writing in the medical journal, *The Practitioner,* in 1972, advised anyone suffering from diverticular disease to have plenty of unrefined food such as wholemeal bread, porridge, fruit and vegetables, but that as such a diet tended to be expensive, he recommended that the cheapest way of replacing the fibre missing in our 'civilized' diet was to add unprocessed bran to the food, up to 4 tablespoons daily until the bowels open once or twice daily without straining. Presumably, once this goal had been achieved the patient was allowed to carry on with the deficient 'civilized' diet, only to set in motion once again the chain of events which had made it necessary to seek the advice of the 'specialist'.

It is not surprising that some patients who act on this type of advice and bulk up their deficient diet with large doses of indigestible fibrous material should be plagued with flatulence and abdominal distension as a result of increasing the metabolic burdens imposed on an already weakened digestive system.

So once again it is necessary to stress the overriding principle which *must* be accepted and acted upon by all who seek to regain or retain bodily health but which still seems to be ignored or denied by all but an enlightened few members of the medical establishment: optimum nutrition can only be achieved by consuming moderate amounts of simple whole foods which contain all the essential nutrients in their natural state and proper proportions. Once the vital nutritional balance of a staple food has been changed or destroyed by commercial processing and chemical manipulation it cannot be restored by subsequent 'reinforcement' with synthetic substitutes; nor can the deficiencies be made good by supplementation with concentrated, extracted and perhaps synthesized vitamins and minerals. For all their wizardry, the 'nutritional chemists' can never produce a nutrient substance which has the same *qualitative* characteristics as those which are fashioned by nature.

Water

We have now reviewed the more important 'dry goods' which are transported through the alimentary canal via the various staging posts, but there remains another essential nutrient to which little or no thought is given by either the nutritional experts or the general public – namely water.

It is a surprising fact that water in one form or another constitutes more than 60 per cent of the bodily tissues and that this fluid is changed and replaced constantly, either by the beverages that are consumed or by the fluid content of the foods we eat. It is estimated that in order to maintain this vital fluid balance the average person living in a temperate climate needs to take in approximately 2¾ litres (5 pints) of liquid daily in order to make good that which is excreted through the eliminative organs. Rather more than 50 per cent, after being filtered through the kidneys, is passed as urine, a further 25 per cent is lost through the skin in the form of perspiration, some 20 per cent is passed from the lungs as vapour in the breath, and the remaining small percentage is excreted from the bowel in the faeces. These quantities and proportions can, of course, vary quite considerably under certain circumstances, such as in very hot climates when the loss through perspiration can reach an astonishing 8¼ litres (15 pints).

Only when these facts are realized can we appreciate that the nature and quality of the beverages we drink are as important to bodily well-being as the other substances which are channelled through the alimentary canal. It is probable, however, that very few of those who live in Western communities habitually drink the natural spring water which Nature has provided for our well-being, and that only very rarely do we drink to satisfy true thirst or, indeed, eat only to appease true hunger.

Eating and drinking are indulged in by most of us as a social or domestic ritual, and just as we eat regularly at fixed mealtimes each day, regardless of our physiological needs for sustenance, so we have become habituated to taking frequent cups of tea or coffee or glasses of milk, beer, wine, spirits, synthetic

'fruit' squashes and other dubious commercial concoctions, many of which contain potentially harmful
chemical substances and few of which have any real
nutritive properties. And yet these are the fluids which
we pour, unthinkingly, into our alimentary canal and
which compound the other gastronomic abuses which
are imposed on the stomach, kidneys, liver and
intestines.

It is an undeniable fact that many of the foods and
beverages which are consumed today are coloured,
preserved, flavoured and doctored in innumerable
ways with the products of the chemical laboratory, and
are also processed, cooked and de-natured to such an
extent that the end-products are virtually devoid of
nutritional value. It is not surprising, therefore, that the
body's ability to maintain vital tissues and functions is
steadily eroded and that eventual breakdown of the
sensitive and highly specialized digestive, assimilative
and eliminative organs which constitute the alimentary
canal should become almost inevitable, leading to the
alarming increase in the incidence of peptic ulceration,
colitis and diverticulitis. There can be little doubt, also,
that failure by the orthodox medical profession to
recognize the fundamental nutritional causes of these
degenerative diseases, and their reliance on suppressive and harmful drugs in an effort to allay the troublesome symptoms, is a major factor in the ever-increasing
number of deaths from cancer.

Only when we accept the logic of identifying and removing the *causes* of organic breakdown and functional failure can we have any hope of restoring and maintaining optimum health.

4

Diverticulitis – its symptoms and causes

The medical term, 'diverticulitis', means inflammation of a diverticulum. The latter word – being derived from the Latin terms 'di', meaning 'aside', and 'vert˘ere', meaning 'to turn' – is applied to a condition in which food residues in the large intestine are 'turned aside' into small pouches or sacs which form in the walls of the bowel as a result of abnormal pressure and distension. In time, the trapped material may ferment and putrefy, causing the damaged mucous membranes to become inflamed, hence 'diverticulitis'.

The development of diverticulae, a condition termed diverticulosis, has become increasingly common since the middle years of the twentieth century, particularly among people over middle age. In the early stages of the disorder few if any symptoms may be experienced, although there is likely to be a history of constipation alternating perhaps with occasional bouts of diarrhoea. Increasingly frequent attacks of abdominal discomfort and distension will be experienced which may be ascribed to indigestion due to unwise eating.

When, however, as is largely inevitable, inflammation supervenes the patient will experience increasing and more continuous abdominal discomfort and tenderness and there may be some degree of fever accompanied by muscular rigidity over the area of the lesion. In severe and long-standing cases an abscess may form in one or more of the diverticulae. If such a lesion should perforate, serious complications will arise in the form of bowel obstruction and peritonitis, and adjacent organs such as the bladder and vagina may become involved. At this stage surgical intervention may become unavoidable.

When, as is rarely the case, the bowel disorder occurs in infancy it will be due to a congenital defect and here, again, recourse to surgery is likely to be necessary. Where, however, the symptoms arise later in life it is important that a reliable diagnosis is established as soon as possible. The more sophisticated X-ray techniques which are now available, allied to a greater awareness of the possible implications of the early symptoms, makes it possible to take effective corrective measures before the degenerative changes in the tissues of the bowel wall have become too advanced and irreversible.

Except in the very worst cases, however, it is often possible to put into effect what may be termed 'holding operations', to strengthen the weakened tissues, and promote more efficient bowel function. This, in turn, guards against the build-up of putrefying material in the diverticulae which may cause the increasing congestion and inflammation leading eventually to ulceration.

At whatever stage the symptoms have reached when diverticulosis or diverticulitis is diagnosed the first priority must be to gain a clear understanding of the nature of the problem and the various factors which, possibly over a fairly considerable period, have led to its development.

Orthodox medical treatment

Even a cursory study of modern medical literature, whether it be a clinical text-book or one of the popular 'home doctor' publications, will reveal that there is a unanimous acceptance of the fact that long-standing constipation is a common denominator in virtually every case of diverticular disease. Consequently it is seen that a diet lacking in vegetable fibre is a major predisposing factor in regard to the impaired bowel function.

As was mentioned briefly in the preceding chapter, this represents a complete 'about-face' in medical thinking with regard to the causes of bowel disorders generally. It also marks a reversal in their approach to treatment, since as recently as the middle-years of the twentieth century, sufferers were being assured that their dietary habits had little or nothing to do with their health problems and they were being advised to avoid all fibrous foods and rely on doses of liquid paraffin and other purgatives to stimulate peristalsis in the weakened bowel.

Even when, in the late 1960s and early 1970s, the enlightened research work of a few surgeons and doctors, notably T. L. Cleave, N. S. Painter and D. P. Burkitt, demonstrated beyond doubt that the low-residue diet was actually responsible for the bowel stasis which was the precursor of diverticulosis and other intestinal disorders, the medical profession generally still resisted the naturopathic assertion that a radical change in dietary habits is essential if a lasting solution to such problems is to be achieved.

Instead, they simply advised their patients to take large doses of bran daily while allowing them to continue to eat the refined and de-natured foods which, over the years, had caused their bowel problems. In other words, they remained totally committed to the 'remedy mentality' and simply prescribed bran as they would any other form of medication, ignoring the basic dietetic causes and simply attempting to banish the symptom.

Naturopaths maintain that it is precisely this attitude which has been very largely responsible for the increasing incidence of chronic bowel disorders, such as diverticular disease, ulcerative colitis and even cancer of the colon for which, ultimately, major surgery is necessary. The number of patients who are being subjected to this operation, termed colostomy, represents a graphic indication of the failure of orthodox treatment of acute bowel disorders and the need for a radical change in the medical assessment of symptoms and their significance.

It is not sufficient simply to note the nature of the systemic or organic malfunction of which a patient complains, enquire about the type of pain or discomfort and its location, and perhaps arrange for tests to be carried out before giving the condition a label such as constipation, flatulence, irritable colon, etc. Even then followers of orthodox treatments may merely prescribe medicine, pills or tablets, and tell the patient to report back for another prescription in a week or two if there is no improvement?

As we shall explain in the next chapter, all that can be achieved by such treatment is the relief – or more correctly the *suppression* – of the patient's symptoms while ignoring what is surely the self-evident fact that pain, discomfort and malfunction are nature's warning signs that something is amiss. Such short-sightedness is akin to switching off a fire alarm and doing nothing about the fire.

An alternative approach

The naturopathic approach, on the other hand, is to assess all the patient's symptoms and then delve into the details of his or her diet, habits, activities and previous health history in order to identify the errors of omission and commission which could have been in anyway responsible for the present problems. Armed with this detailed assessment, it is possible to begin the process of re-education and adjustment which will remove or correct whatever activities are suspected of causing the symptoms, so allowing the body to mobilize its very efficient self-healing powers and rebuild damaged tissues and restore functional and organic health.

It must surely be self-evident that a condition such as diverticulitis does not develop suddenly or even in the course of a few months. The human body has a tremendous capacity to withstand abuse and misuse, and it has a remarkable ability to adapt its complex functions and systems in order to neutralize the effects of potentially harmful habits and practices. It would, therefore, be totally unrealistic to expect to be able to correct or even minimize the effects of tissue breakdown and organic dysfunction simply by taking a medicinal concoction for a few weeks or, in the case of diverticulitis, sprinkling some bran over one's food.

The formation of diverticulae represents the end-result of long-standing stress, not only on the tissues of the colon itself but on all the other complex systems and organs which constitute the alimentary canal. It may have had its earliest origins in childhood or adolescence when, as a result of parental ignorance or financial stringency, much of the diet consisted of white-flour concoctions coupled with peeled and boiled or fried vegetables and tinned or packeted convenience foods, all of which had been deprived of their natural fibrous elements and much of their normal nutritional value. They may also have been coloured, flavoured, and treated in various other ways with potentially toxic chemical additives. Such a diet would have posed many problems for the digestive and eliminative organs, but the inbuilt capacity for adaptation and tolerance may well have staved off its more serious consequences. This would be particularly so if the individual concerned was maintaining a reasonably high degree of general fitness by engaging regularly in physical activities, such as strenuous games and sports.

It is likely, however, that the false sense of security thus engendered will be rudely shattered when, in later years, domestic and occupational demands reduce the amount of time that can be spared for such indulgences. Sooner or later the acquisition of a car eventually obviates even the need for such mundane activities as walking to the station, shops or bus-stop. Moreover, the almost universal addiction to television means that it will no longer be necessary to stir from the armchair in order to watch one's favourite sports or to visit a cinema or theatre.

The overall effects of these radical changes in our feeding and physical habits has taken an inevitable toll on the systems and organs which comprise the alimentary canal. Dietary deficiencies and excesses disorganize the chemical structure of the secretions on which the complex processes of digestion and absorption are dependent, and clutter up the intestines with a slow-moving mass of incompletely digested food residues. The result is to steadily increase congestion in the abdominal organs and distend and weaken the muscles which surround and support them, muscles which have already been weakened as a result of physical inactivity.

The combination of faulty nutrition and sedentary habits leads almost inevitably to some degree of bowel stasis for the relief of which recourse may be had to a laxative which, at best, may afford some degree of temporary relief. The fallacy of this treatment, however, is that laxatives and purgatives are substances which have irritant properties and so they stimulate the muscular tissues in the bowel walls into activity by goading them into spasms of peristaltic activity and causing the glands in the irritated bowel walls to secrete a copious flow of mucus. In effect, they precipitate a form of diarrhoea so that the liquefied food residues are excreted rapidly and forcibly. The patient is lulled into the belief that his or her problem has been effectively solved, but since nothing has been done to correct the underlying causes of the bowel congestion and weakness it *must* be only a matter of time before the same train of events recurs. Thus, a vicious circle is established: constipation, → irritant purgation,→ diarrhoea. Each time the congested bowel is spurred into activity it becomes weaker and less responsive to the irritant substance and so the dosage has to be increased until a point is reached where the muscles and membranes can no longer cope with the demands imposed upon them.

This, it must be conceded, is an extreme example of the chain of events which leads to the breakdown of the bowel walls and the formation of diverticulae, but whether bodily abuses are compounded so dramatically or are imposed in lesser degree over a period of years, the causes of the ultimate breakdown are basically the same.

The far-reaching consequences

It is necessary to digress at this point to explain that the same factors which, in some individuals, cause bowel and digestive disorders, may have even more serious implications in regard to other aspects of bodily health. The implications involve such vital organs as the heart, arteries, liver and kidneys, the functional efficiency of which is equally dependent upon nutritional balance and physical fitness. Those who have even a vague recollection of school biology lessons will know that when food has been digested the nutrients which it contained are absorbed through the bowel walls into the bloodstream and transported via the arteries and veins, directly or indirectly, to those organs and tissues where they are needed for growth or repair or to provide heat and energy. What is perhaps less widely appreciated is the potentially harmful effects of physical inactivity on the efficiency of the vital transport system.

The prime mover in the circulatory system is the heart, which is basically a powerful, muscular pump, primed with freshly oxygenated blood from the lungs which is then propelled to all parts of the body via the arteries. Having delivered oxygen and nutrients to the various tissues and organs and taken up waste products, the blood is then returned to the heart through a vast network of capillaries and veins. At this stage, however, the pumping effect of the heart has been dissipated and in order to propel the blood on its return journey, much of it against the downward pull of gravity, the body relies on the auxiliary pumping effect produced by the alternate contraction and relaxation of the muscles surrounding the veins. The latter are provided with an ingenious system of valves which prevent any reflux flow of the blood when pressure from the muscles is relaxed.

Therefore, any activity such as walking, jogging, swimming, rowing or climbing stairs which entails rhythmic movement of the arms and legs will not only activate what has been described appropriately as the 'muscle-pump', but also initiate deep breathing. The resultant contraction and expansion of the lungs combined with the simultaneous raising and lowering of the muscular diaphragm beneath them exerts a powerful suction effect on the large veins passing through the abdomen and so draws the blood upward through the chest cavity and back to the heart. Without this circulatory support the blood tends to form a pool in the lower limbs and abdomen, with the result that tissue nutrition is impaired and cell debris, carbon dioxide and other metabolic wastes cannot be transported to the eliminative organs for disposal.

Here, again, the combination of dietetic errors and lack of exercise is responsible for the circulatory stasis. This, in turn, brings about the congestion which manifests itself in such common disorders as constipation, haemorrhoids (piles) and varicose veins and, eventually, in the potentially more serious degenerative disorders with which we are now concerned, i.e. diverticulosis and diverticulitis.

The effects of stress

In discussing the various factors which combine to weaken the components of the alimentary canal, we should not ignore the effects of mental and emotional stress. It is widely recognized that the human body is capable of responding positively to recurring crises and that an efficient 'flight or fight' reaction to any external threat is an essential component in nature's inbuilt survival mechanism. When a threatening situation arises, alarm bells are triggered off in the brain in response to which all systems are alerted in readiness for whatever action needs to be taken either to combat the threat or to run away from it. The immediate effects are to increase the pulse and respiration rates, raise the blood pressure and divert the blood supply from the digestive organs and surface tissues to the brain, the lungs and the muscles so that the body is ready to react with the utmost speed and efficiency. Only when the crisis is past are the alarm bells switched off and normal services resumed throughout the body.

It is a system which would be of the utmost value to the individual if such emergencies occurred only infrequently and lasted for relatively short periods. Unfortunately 'civilized' man does not live in a 'normal', natural world, and when, as is often the case, business, domestic and economic crises are a source of constant or recurring anxiety and fear, the effects on the digestive system can be quite devastating.

It has already been shown that as food traverses the alimentary canal its digestion and assimilation are dependent on the release of complex chemical secretions at each of the various staging posts (see Chapter 2). Under conditions of stress, however, these secretory processes are suspended, so that the body's resources can be concentrated on resisting the potential threat. A situation of extreme danger will cause the body to react so violently that any food in the stomach will be ejected by vomiting and the contents of the bowel will also be cleared by involuntary defaecation.

When, however, an individual is plagued by a succession of nagging anxieties and worries, the food that he or she consumes remains in the alimentary canal but, because the functions of the secretory glands have been suspended, it will not be properly digested and assimilated. Consequently, a mass of food residues will accumulate in the intestines and so accentuate any existing pressure and congestion which, as we have seen already, are among the contributory factors which lead to the breakdown of the bowel lining and the formation of diverticulae.

An understanding of the effects of stress on bodily health is therefore essential if a co-ordinated course of treatment is to be fully effective.

The crucial role of the lymphatic system

Before we close this chapter there is yet another very important circulatory system which needs to be explained, one of which few people are aware but which, if anything, plays an even more vital role in safeguarding bodily health than that of the blood. This second network of vessels – known as the lymphatic system – ramifies throughout the body in close proximity to the blood vessels. As the blood from the arteries permeates through the network of minute capillaries before being taken up by the veins and returned to the heart, one of its constituents – a clear, watery fluid called lymph – is drawn off into the adjacent lymphatic vessels. The constituents of this fluid are similar to those of the blood plasma. However, whereas the role of the blood is confined mainly to carrying nutrients to the tissue cells, taking up carbon dioxide and helping to seal off wounds, the lymph has the additional function of trapping and destroying harmful bacteria and neutralizing other toxic substances which threaten the body's well-being.

The tiny lymphatic capillaries, like those of the venous system, gradually unite as they carry their vital fluid from the extremities towards the heart, thus forming ever-larger vessels. These eventually empty into two terminal veins in the base of the neck which then return the lymph and blood to the heart for recirculation around the body. Like the veins, the lymphatic vessels depend almost entirely upon the 'muscle-pump' for the propulsion of their contents up through the lower limbs, abdomen and thorax against the downward pull of gravity. Like the veins, also, they are equipped with valves at frequent intervals to prevent reflux.

There is, however, one very important feature which differentiates the lymphatic vessels from the veins, namely, that at strategic points in the system, notably the chest and abdomen but also in the vicinity of the main joints such as the knees, groins, elbows, armpits and beneath the chin, the lymphatics pass through groups of lymph glands or nodes. It is here that any bacteria and other potentially harmful substances are filtered out of the lymph and destroyed by masses of specialized white blood corpuscles called leucocytes. The leucocytes are concentrated in the lymph glands for this specific purpose, their numbers being greatly augmented when the need arises to cope with crises such as serious infection or a septic wound. The operation of this vital defence mechanism becomes readily apparent when the glands in the neck become enlarged and hardened during a bout of tonsillitis say, or when those under the arm swell up due to an injury to the hand turning septic or a boil erupting nearby.

Even this brief description of the circulation demonstrates that lack of physical exercise not only predisposes to abdominal weakness and congestion, but also reduces the efficiency of the muscle-pump, with the result that maintenance and repair of the tissues of the colon are impaired by stagnation of the blood supply and toxic wastes and bacteria cannot be effectively neutralized and destroyed by the lymphatic system. The resultant vicious circle can only be broken if the sufferer from diverticulitis appreciates fully the relevance of physical exercise in the treatment of diverticular disease and is prepared to carry out, patiently and conscientiously, the *full* programme of remedial measures set out in Chapter 8.

It also helps to make clear why, as no doubt some of the readers of this book have discovered for themselves, orthodox medical treatment of bowel disorders has not only failed to afford more than some measure of temporary relief of the painful symptoms, but in many cases has allowed the condition to become progressively more troublesome. We shall elaborate more fully on the reasons for this frustrating state of affairs in the next chapter.

5

Medical myopia

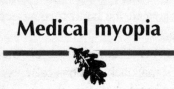

Articles in the press and other branches of the media, usually written by so-called 'medical correspondents' who seldom have any formal medical qualifications, frequently repeat the claim that 'advances in medical science' are responsible for the conquest of diseases such as smallpox, diphtheria, scarlet fever, and so on which were rife in the early years of the twentieth century. A similar claim is often made in respect of the increased expectancy of life today as compared with that of earlier generations. The fact is, however, that most of the credit for these achievements belongs, not to the medical profession, but to the very considerable improvements in public hygiene and living standards which have come about since the turn of the century.

For example, the decline in deaths attributable to smallpox had started well before the introduction of compulsory vaccination, and the disease is virtually unknown today despite the fact that the vaccination of infants has long since ceased to be mandatory. Similarly, the average life-expectancy of men and women over the age of 50 has changed very little over the same period of time, and such apparent improvements as have been claimed are due almost exclusively to the very marked reduction in infant mortality brought about by improved social conditions.

There is, indeed, no possible justification for describing the practice of medicine as a science, since that term implies that its methods are demonstrably based on irrefutable and unchangeable fact, whereas anyone who reviews even the recent history of medicine will realize that what is claimed as sound practice at one time is discredited and discarded only a decade or two later.

This is in no sense a criticism of the individual practitioner who, in the vast majority of cases, practises conscientiously *what he or she has been taught*. Regrettably, however, modern medical practice is overwhelmingly drug-orientated, and during the long and arduous training which the medical student undergoes the emphasis is almost exclusively on medication. He is required to have a detailed understanding of human anatomy and physiology, and to learn complex diagnostic techniques and the signs and symptoms of disease, but throughout the course the recurring theme is the prescription of specific drugs for each specific disease entity. He or she knows that in order to graduate it will be necessary to give answers in the final examinations which accord with the material disseminated by the tutors and gleaned from the text-books approved by medical hierarchy. The same kind of indoctrination will continue throughout the time he or she is required to serve as a junior practitioner in hospitals where, under the eyes of his seniors, he will be expected to adhere strictly to established medical practices and principles.

When, eventually, he is able to take his place in general practice, probably as a junior member of a busy team of GPs, the demands of surgery sessions and house calls will leave him little time to do more than conduct a hasty consultation with each patient, ask a few questions and perhaps carry out a very brief examination before appending a label to the ailment and scribbling a prescription for the drug of his choice. Once caught up in such an exacting routine it is likely that he will have little time to question the validity of what he is doing, and since a large proportion of the symptoms with which he is confronted are likely to be self-limiting, he may justifiably have no cause or inclination to do so.

The power of the drug companies

Indeed, the doctor is actively discouraged from questioning what he is doing by the drug manufacturers who bombard him with samples of their products and glossy literature lauding the therapeutic virtues of their latest drugs. Significantly, it is invariably claimed that these are more effective and have fewer harmful side-effects than their own earlier 'wonder drugs' or those of their competitors.

Nor do the blandishments of the drug companies stop at the dissemination of advertising propaganda supported often by a personal call from a persuasive sales representative. In addition, if his professional status is sufficiently high, a generous gift may be left on his desk or he may even be invited to join other eminent practitioners at a luxurious hotel or holiday resort for an expenses-paid 'conference' or 'seminar', where every opportunity will be taken to press home the virtues of the host's products. A report published in the 1980s claimed that the drug industry was spending no less than £5,000 on each GP in order to promote its proprietary medicines.

It is not surprising, therefore, that having established such a firm stranglehold on the medical profession, the pharmaceutical industry is dominated by some of the largest and wealthiest multi-national companies. The rapidly increasing turn-over and growth of such companies should be a cause for concern to all except those who run them and the shareholders who see their investments and dividends soaring from year to year. For despite the fact that expenditure on drugs and the financial burden which it imposes on the so-called National Health Service continue to escalate year by year, there has been no reciprocal improvement in the overall health of the general public.

When, in 1948, Aneurin Bevan founded the NHS he envisaged a future in which the provision of comprehensive health care for everyone, regardless of means, would gradually reduce the incidence of disease so that the annual cost of the service would fall progressively. His dream of a nation in which fewer people would require medical attention, spending on the NHS would fall progressively and productivity in industry would be increased as a consequence, has long since turned into a nightmare. Fortunately, he did not live to see the cost of his idealistic scheme rocket to become a multi-million-pound millstone round the neck of the national exchequer and be estimated to have become the world's largest employer except for the Soviet military authorities.

The fact is that what Nye Bevan intended to be a National *Health* Service has, over the years, deteriorated into a National *Medical* Service which, instead of seeking to improve the health of the people and prevent illness, is content merely to issue many millions of prescriptions annually for ever more potent drugs which themselves cause often unpredictable and serious side-effects, some of which are worse than the disease symptoms they were meant to 'cure'.

The harmful side-effects of modern drugs

A standard medical pharmacopoeia on which doctors rely for information regarding the medicines and pills that they prescribe consists of more than 2,000 pages of very small print. It lists a vast number of drugs and explains both their specific uses and the harmful effects to which they are known to give rise. There is, in fact, a specialist body which has been set up for the sole purpose of monitoring drug-induced diseases and to which doctors are required to report any untoward reaction which occurs in patients undergoing treatment.

It is not only naturopaths and other drugless practitioners who have warned of the dangers of prescription mania. A London University Professor of Psychology blamed drug companies for not recognizing the problems that their drugs could cause and claimed that some people were being admitted to hospital simply because they had been so poisoned by a build-up of drugs that they could no longer look after themselves. He was particularly concerned about the tens of thousands of old people who, he maintained, are 'hooked' on medically prescribed tranquillizers and sleeping tablets such as valium, librium and mogadon. As a result of addiction the 'geriatric junkies', as he called them, may suffer from a variety of symptoms such as sweating, nausea, loss of concentration, confusion and anti-social behaviour which may lead to a false diagnosis and result in their being prescribed even larger doses of the drugs.

Another London doctor, writing in a national news-paper, admitted that medical practitioners are guilty of poisoning many of their patients with drugs that are not required and which are sometimes dangerous. He claimed that between 5 and 10 per cent of all hospital admissions are due to doctor-induced disease. Every year, he said, three million unnecessary prescriptions are issued for antibiotics, a claim which is of special significance in regard to diverticulitis and other bowel disorders. In Chapter 2 it was shown how the beneficial bacteria inhabit the healthy intestines and play a very important part in the digestive processes, in addition to manufacturing certain components of the vitamin B complex. The destructive effect of an antibiotic on these bacteria is catastrophic, and as a result the efficiency of the digestive and assimilative systems will be impaired for some considerable time following a course of treatment with a drug of this kind.

Nor is it only the more sophisticated prescription medicines that play a part in disrupting the complex functions of the alimentary canal. Even a simple household remedy such as aspirin, many millions of which are taken annually for the relief of common ailments, is now known to be highly irritant to the mucous membranes which line the digestive tract. Indeed, one of the foremost pharmaceutical reference books devotes more than four closely printed pages to these harmful side-effects, their treatment and the precautions which doctors are advised to observe when prescribing the drug:

> An important toxic effect which may occur even with small doses [of aspirin] is irritation of the gastric mucosa and resultant dyspepsia, erosion, ulceration, haematemesis and melaena [bleeding]; slight blood loss may occur in about 70% of patients with most aspirin preparations, whether buffered, soluble or plain.

There is little doubt, as we have already indicated, that resorting to the use of laxatives in an effort to relieve constipation is another important factor in the geneses of diverticulitis. The same pharmaceutical reference work quoted above devotes some ten pages to the various drugs prescribed for this purpose. To their credit, the compilers warn that:

> the constant use of purgatives to induce a daily habit, which is commonly believed to be necessary for good

health, may decrease the sensitivity of the intestinal mucous membranes so that larger doses have to be taken and the bowel fails to respond to normal stimuli. Thus the re-development of a normal habit is prevented.

Unfortunately, a vast quantity of proprietary laxatives is purchased by the public direct from chemists and other retail outlets and no such health warning is printed on the labels of these products. Unless, therefore, the purchaser has been warned of the potential dangers of the laxative habit, the progressive deterioration of the bowel function and eventual degeneration of its tissues is almost inevitable.

There can be other hazards also, since no drug is entirely free from harmful side-effects. There are many examples in medical history of drugs which are deemed to be safe after extensive laboratory tests, only to be withdrawn subsequently as a result of the very serious and even fatal effects on patients which come to light after they have been widely prescribed. Two in particular, which have attracted world-wide publicity, are Opren and Thalidomide. The former was the cause of serious illness and death in patients taking the drug for the relief of arthritis, while the latter resulted in the birth of thousands of babies with terrible deformities after their mothers were prescribed the tranquillizer during pregnancy.

Less dramatic, but more specifically relevant to readers of this book, is the fact that liquid paraffin, which was very widely used for the relief of constipation, was found not only to cause damage to the tissues of the intestines but also to prevent the absorption into the bloodstream of the fat-soluble vitamins A and D. There were reports, also, of cases of pneumonia occurring in patients who had become dependent on the laxative.

Much more could be written to underline the folly and futility of the orthodox medical approach of trying to solve the problems of acute and chronic illnesses simply by the use of drugs and/or by procedures which suppress or relieve symptoms but do nothing to remove or correct the faulty nutritional and other factors which allow disease conditions to develop in the first place. It is hoped, however, that enough has been explained to enable the reader to understand the true nature and causes of diverticular disease. And that this, in turn, allows them to recognize the logic of the naturopathic approach to the problem and so be prepared to carry out conscientiously and confidently the full programme of tissue-cleansing and reconstructive measures which alone will relieve bowel inflammation and congestion and allow the body's remarkably efficient self-healing powers to repair the damaged tissues and restore normal, healthy function.

6

The road to recovery

W e make no apology for having dealt at such length with the many obstructive and destructive influences which, in combination and often over a period of many years, disorganize the vital functions of the alimentary canal, weaken its tissues and cause the kind of breakdown which allows diverticulae to form. Only when these factors are clearly understood will the reader be able to recognize what it is that he or she has done, or left undone, and so opened the way to the predicament with which we are now concerned.

It cannot be reiterated too often that if a satisfactory and lasting solution to these problems is to be achieved it is vital that the reader has a clear understanding not only of *what* needs to be done but – and this is even more important – *why* the various treatment measures are necessary.

The fundamental principle upon which all na-turopathic treatment is based is that the human body has a near-miraculous capacity for tissue repair and self-healing which enables it to resolve all but the most advanced disease problems once the necessary conditions and materials are provided. This facility is clearly demonstrated when someone is involved in an accident and sustains broken bones or torn flesh. We all know that with little or no outside interven-tion other than cleansing the wounds and ensuring warmth and rest, the damaged tissues will heal spon-taneously. Precisely the same forces can be called to our aid when internal tissues and organs are damaged, and regeneration will be achieved with the same facility if we ensure that the right conditions are provided.

If, therefore, the damaged bowel lining is to be repaired the first priority is to cleanse the wound by clearing away any obstructing debris which may be causing localized congestion and inflammation. The only logical way to achieve this end is through thera-peutic fasting, meaning withholding unwanted food material for a short period. For many people the idea of going without food voluntarily for any length of time is almost unthinkable. Most of us have been brought up from infancy in the belief that, regardless of circumstances, one *must*, at all times, continue to eat in order to 'keep up one's strength'. This is just one more manifestation of the medical myopia to which we have already referred. It is exemplified by the way patients in hospital are constantly pressurized into taking some form of food, either liquid or solid, no matter what their illness may be, and even though they may have no desire to eat. Indeed, the very sight or smell of food may evoke revulsion in some circumstances.

Those who insist on what amounts to forced feeding fail to recognize that the partial or total loss of appetite is the expression of the natural instinct which all other living creatures obey when faced with illness or injury. Anyone who has owned a cat or a dog will know that under such circumstances even a domesticated animal will 'go off its food' and ignore all efforts to tempt it to eat, even when offered delicacies a healthy pet would find irresistible. Instead, the animals will usually seek out a warm secluded place to sleep or rest undisturbed, taking nothing more than an occasional drink of water. Only when they are well on the way to recovery will they begin to take solid food and return gradually to normal activity.

Why, then, do we, as intelligent and reasoning beings, defy this natural instinct? An instinct which clearly insists that our ailing digestive system needs to be rested to allow the self-healing and rebuilding resources to be mobilized and to function efficiently as nature intended? What possible justification can there be for flouting a primary instinct for self-preservation and allowing ourselves to be persuaded by well-meaning but misguided doctors or relatives to take not only unwanted food but also potentially harmful drugs which can only increase the burdens on our already weakened digestive and metabolic systems and at best delay, and at worst prevent, recovery?

The only possible – though totally illogical – answer to these questions is that we have become so habituated to the daily ritual of eating at fixed mealtimes, regardless of physiological needs, that we cannot contemplate the thought of voluntarily abstaining from food for even one day. The suggestion that such nutritional deprivation should be continued for two or even three days must, therefore seem to be quite unthinkable and fraught with the direst consequences.

Step one: Fasting

It is true that the instinct to fast is felt most strongly at the onset of *acute* illnesses such as fevers and other inflammatory and congestive conditions. When such disorders are treated by suppressive medication instead of being allowed to resolve themselves naturally, what we term 'appetite' will gradually return. However, if as often happens under these circumstances, the patient develops a chronic illness the instinctive reaction becomes progressively weakened, and the body's ability to respond to abuse and misuse is gradually eroded. The fact that at this stage the weakened organism has lost its capacity to sound the alarm signals in no way invalidates the naturopathic principle that rest and tissue-cleansing procedures are essential prerequisites if the self-healing and repairing processes are to be mobilized efficiently. Hence the need for a short period of voluntary fasting.

It is relevant to point out at this stage that there are millions of people throughout the world who regularly undertake fasts of varying duration for religious and other reasons and who consider themselves to be physically and spiritually uplifted as a result. The fact that therapeutic fasting, as advocated by the naturopathic movement for more than a century, is widely misunderstood in Western communities is due largely to misrepresentation by the orthodox medical profession and the popular media. Both of these have instilled an element of fear in the minds of the public by implying that fasting is synonymous with starvation. There is, however, no possible foundation for any such misapprehension. The emaciated limbs, bloated abdomen and sunken cheeks of the victims of true starvation, which regrettably have become all too familiar through the television documentaries depicting the results of prolonged famine in some Third World communities, can in no way be equated with the minor physical changes which take place in patients during a relatively short period of therapeutic fasting. Indeed, very protracted periods of fasting have been employed successfully and safely by naturopaths, under careful supervision in residential clinics, for the treatment of chronically sick patients.

Although the obvious physical effects of a short fast may be no more than the loss of a certain amount of often superfluous weight, the physiological effects can be far-reaching and of very considerable therapeutic benefit. It can be stated with complete confidence that nothing but good can result from a short fast of three or four days carried out carefully by a patient who is well-informed as to the nature and purpose of the procedure and who has sufficient confidence and resolution to ignore any well-meaning but misguided doubts and fears which may be voiced by friends or relatives. There is no therapeutic procedure which affords a more efficient means of stimulating into action the tissue-cleansing processes which constitute an essential preliminary to the healing and reconstructive measures triggered by cleaning the bowel of the accumulation of fermenting residues. It is these residues that are responsible for the inflammation and congestion which cause the breakdown in the walls of the colon. Moreover, once we cease to burden the digestive organs with unwanted food we release vital energy which can then be directed towards restoration and repair.

Step two: a healing diet

Having relieved the bowel of the burden of debris we can then proceed to soothe the inflamed mucous membranes by means of a carefully chosen diet of fresh fruits together with drinks of dilute fruit and vegetable juices. The alkaline properties of the latter serve to dilute and neutralize any potentially irritant acids which may be released by the over-sensitive secretory glands. At the same time we shall be supplying vitamins and other nutrients together with sufficient fibrous bulk to stimulate a gentle peristaltic action and so further facilitate the cleansing process.

Thus, as the various components of the alimentary canal are coaxed into renewed action, essential nutrients are once again released into the bloodstream and made available for the repair of damaged tissues. At the same time any discarded cell wastes and unwanted food residues will be disposed of promptly and efficiently.

The next phase of the treatment involves increasing the variety and quantity of wholesome but easily digested foods so that the digestive and eliminative organs are encouraged to process a greater variety of nutrient materials. Initially this will entail having frequent small meals of simple whole foods. These should be eaten slowly and masticated thoroughly so that they can be mixed with the various digestive secretions and processed efficiently as they pass through the staging posts in the alimentary canal. For this purpose, fruits and vegetables constitute the bulk of the diet, but to avoid imposing unnecessary strain on the digestive organs most of the food will be cooked lightly. This should ensure that there is the least possible damage to vitamins and other nutrients some of which are susceptible to excessive or prolonged heat. Neither salt nor sugar should be added to these foods either during cooking or at the table.

It must be emphasized that nothing but small amounts of what are termed alkaline foods – fruits and vegetables – may be taken during this transitionary period following the short fast. However, once this phase has been completed it becomes possible for the digestive system to accept and process an amplified and balanced diet which will provide the body with all the essential nutrients needed to restore its organs and tissues to full functional efficiency.

At this stage it is relevant to explain that what are sometimes referred to as 'acid fruits' do, in fact, have an alkaline reaction as a result of the chemical processes to which they are subjected during digestion. The foods which are largely responsible for what is often referred to as 'acid indigestion' or 'acidity' are the sugars, proteins and starches, especially when the latter are derived from white flour, polished rice and other refined cereals. It is for this reason that the diet which we shall advocate once the cleansing and transitional stages of treatment have been completed will consist of approximately 60 per cent of the alkaline fruits, vegetables and salads, and not more than 20 per cent each of the acid-forming carbohydrates and proteins. As we have explained in a previous chapter, fats in their pure, extracted form need have little or no place in a properly balanced diet since the body's very limited needs in this respect will be met adequately by the fat content of other foods.

Provided that a reasonably close approximation of the 60:20:20 balance is maintained it will provide all the vitamins, minerals, proteins and carbohydrates – including fibre – in their natural form and combinations, bearing in mind that nutritional *quality* is the overriding consideration in the choice of foods and that *moderation* should be exercised in regard to the quantity which is consumed.

We have referred briefly in a previous chapter to the popular fallacy that meat is an essential component of a healthy diet. Now that we are outlining the therapeutic approach to diverticular disease it is necessary to expand further on this very much misunderstood subject.

Many naturopaths maintain that, far from being health-promoting, meat and other foods derived from animal sources should be eaten, if at all, only in the strictest moderation and that for those who are suffering from any kind of illness, and bowel disorders in particular, a mainly vegetarian diet should be adhered to if the speediest possible recovery is to be achieved. They reason that, anatomically and physiologically, the human alimentary tract is equipped primarily for the digestion of non-animal foods such as seeds, nuts, fruits and vegetables. Our main teeth, for example, are short and flat-surfaced and are designed to *grind* the foods we eat, whereas those of cats, dogs and other carnivores are long, sharp and pointed to enable them to tear flesh from the bones of their prey and swallow it with very little mastication.

They point out, also, that the digestive secretions of carnivorous animals are much more strongly acid than ours and so are better adapted for the rapid breakdown and assimilation of flesh and bone. Finally, and perhaps the most important factor, it is a fact that these animals have a substantially shorter intestinal system, which means that food residues are excreted more rapidly. Because of these differences, when animal products constitute a major part of the human diet, they are not so rapidly broken down and absorbed and the residues pass only slowly along the very much longer intestinal system where they tend, as a result, to ferment and so cause the mucous membranes to become inflamed. Moreover, even in medical circles there is a growing suspicion that the increasing incidence in Western communities of a number of serious organic diseases, such as kidney failure, high blood pressure and coronary heart disease, is linked to the relatively high consumption of flesh foods and animal fats.

Step three: exercising

It is also becoming increasingly clear that lack of physical exercise is another factor which predisposes to these degenerative conditions – yet one more fact which has been proclaimed by naturopaths for many decades and which is now being hailed as an important medical breakthrough in the fight against disease. Again, therefore, it is necessary to refer back to an earlier chapter in which we explained the part played by the circulatory and lymphatic systems (see Chapter 4). This showed how these systems distributed nutrient materials to tissues and organs throughout the body and removed carbon dioxide and other toxic materials, while neutralizing or destroying harmful bacteria. Reiteration is necessary in order to impress upon the reader why physical activity and remedial exercises must form an integral part of any comprehensive treatment programme. Without the effective support of the 'muscle-pump' it is not possible to relieve abdominal congestion, restore efficient peristalsis and promote the efficient blood and lymph circulation which is essential if we are to cleanse and repair damaged intestinal tissues.

The special exercises which are outlined later (see Appendix A) are designed primarily to strengthen weakened abdominal muscles and, in combination with dietary measures, reduce any distension in that area. However, it is important that they are complemented by regular outdoor exercise in order to activate the muscle-pump and ensure that the body's self-healing and repair facilities are fully mobilized. For this purpose there is nothing more effective than a brisk walk combined with deep breathing, undertaken as a regular daily discipline and gradually extended in regard to both vigour and duration to the maximum permitted by physical capacity and domestic and occupational commitments.

It is a demonstrable physiological fact that muscular strength and stamina develop in direct proportion to the demands which we impose upon ourselves, which is why it is so essential that remedial exercises and outdoor activity should become an integral part of the therapeutic programme. Care must, of course, be taken in the early stages to avoid undue strain on muscles which may have been weakened by years of sedentary living. This is why walking is by far the best form of exercise for all ages, regardless of sex or physical characteristics. Its great therapeutic value lies in the fact that it involves virtually the whole muscular system – the arms, legs, buttocks, chest, back and shoulders. When it is complemented by deep breathing the muscular diaphragm is also activated with increased vigour, rising and falling with each breath so that blood and lymph are drawn up from the legs and thighs, through the large veins in the abdomen and back to the lungs and heart. The muscular tissues of the heart are strengthened and become progressively more efficient as a result of the demands made upon them. This, in turn, means they are better able to cope with the stresses of daily life, reducing the risks of coronary disease and heart failure.

It will be appreciated, therefore, that the benefits which accrue from regular exercise not just in terms of recovery from a disease such as diverticulitis, but also in terms of better general health and increased life-expectancy must far outweigh any difficulty or inconvenience involved in making the necessary adjustments in one's daily commitments.

Older readers who are retired but who are still physically active should have little difficulty in making available the necessary time. If the walk or other exercise is undertaken as an invariable discipline at a fixed time it should soon become a habitual and enjoyable part of the day's activities, regardless of all but the most severe weather conditions. A pair of good walking shoes or boots is a valuable adjunct, as also is light-weight, windproof clothing in the form of a hooded anorak and waterproof trousers, such as are favoured by ramblers, golfers, etc. They can be purchased at quite reasonable cost from sports outfitters.

Younger people, who have less flexible domestic or occupational commitments and who depend on public transport or the family car for journeys to shops or place of employment, should try to adjust their timetables so that they leave the bus, train or car some distance from their destination and complete the journey on foot, reversing the procedure when returning home. A similar arrangement can perhaps be adopted when visiting shops or friends or taking children to school.

With patience and perseverance it should be possible to make whatever adjustments are required to established habits and routines, bearing in mind the inestimable dividends that will be earned in terms of improving health.

Summary

These, then, are the main components of the therapeutic régime which we shall be employing as a means of solving the problem of diverticular disease:

Step one: A short period of fasting to remove bowel obstructions and relieve congestion, followed by a further brief period of dietary restriction to reduce inflammation.

Step two: The adoption of a balanced, wholefood régime to provide the nutrients needed for the repair and subsequent mainte-nance of tissues and organs.

Step three: A co-ordinated programme of exercises to strengthen the supporting muscles and stimulate the blood and lymph circulatory systems.

Now the time has come to show how these measures are to be co-ordinated into a cohesive programme of effective self-treatment.

7

Prepare for action!

I t cannot be stressed too strongly that maximum benefit from the treatment which we are about to prescribe will only be obtained if the reader has a clear understanding of the nature and purpose of each therapeutic procedure. It is imperative, therefore, that any uncertainty in this respect should be allayed before the commencement of treatment and we would urge that where necessary the preceding chapters should be read and reread.

The initial fasting

The most important step along the road to recovery consists of total abstinence for a few days from *all* solid food, as well as food beverages such as soups, gruels and milk. Stimulants in the form of tea, coffee, alcohol and commercial soft drinks should also be excluded. As a result of the short fast the digestive and assimilative organs and systems are rested completely, thus releasing vital energy for the task of cleansing the tissues and fluids and clearing from the alimentary canal any accumulation of potentially harmful residues.

This initial and possibly most exacting stage of the treatment schedule should be timed to coincide with a period of at least three or four days, and preferably a week or more, when business and domestic demands can be kept to a minimum while the amounts of rest and relaxation can be maximized. Here, again, it is likely that retired and perhaps some self-employed people will be able to make the necessary adjustments without too much difficulty. Others, with occupational or domestic responsibilities may be able to commence treatment just prior to a week-end or take a short holiday, particularly if the help of a spouse, relative or friend can be enlisted. The main objective is to ensure the maximum possible freedom from the more demanding daily chores and responsibilities, together with the opportunity to rest during the day, retire early and have up to eight hours of sound sleep.

It is possible that the fast may induce what is termed a 'healing crisis' as the cleansing processes are activated and result in the onset of some of the eliminative reactions which occur in acute feverish illnesses, e.g. cough, sore throat, headache, aching limbs and lassitude. This is why it is advisable to be able to rest and relax as much as possible. In most cases the symptoms, if any, are likely to be quite mild, but in others, especially if there is a long history of frequent catarrhal upsets such as colds and influenza, a more dramatic reaction may occur in the form of raised temperature, profuse perspiration, enlarged glands and coated tongue.

Such reactions are an indication that the process of tissue-cleansing has begun and it is important that no attempt should be made to suppress them because they play an important part in the body's self-healing efforts.

For example, enlarged glands are an indication of stepped-up lymphatic activity, and profuse perspiration and mucus excretion are utilized as a means of cleansing the body of some of the toxic wastes which have been cluttering up its tissues and fluids.

It is understandable that the onset of such symptoms may be misinterpreted by well-meaning relatives or friends who may predict even more dire consequences if the 'cranky' treatment measures are persisted with. However instead of causing concern, the 'healing crisis' should be welcomed as playing a constructive part in the process of recovery.

During the first 24 hours or so after the commencement of treatment it is likely that the body's 'time-clock' will continue to sound the alarm signal at each customary mealtime, but the habit-actuated demand for food must be resisted, although the pangs of false appetite may be allayed by taking half a tumbler of fresh fruit or vegetable juice diluted with an equal quantity of water. Bottled mineral water is preferred during the course of treatment, but if only tap-water is available it should be boiled, to remove chlorine, and then allowed to cool.

At this time it is likely that the desire for fluid will be increased because of the body's need to dissolve and excrete toxins which are released into the bloodstream as part of the cleansing process. Natural thirst will of course signal any such need which should be satisfied by taking further drinks of mineral water or dilute juice.

The fruit diet

By the end of the third day the eliminative activities will probably have completed their task and the fast may then be broken. Avoid the temptation to 'celebrate' by indulging in a large meal, however. Indeed, for a further two or preferably three days only small meals of fresh fruit should be taken increasing both the quantity and variety gradually so as to allow the digestive and assimilative systems to resume their normal functions of sifting out and utilizing essential nutrients and eliminating the unwanted residues.

During this phase of the treatment it is best to avoid the more acid citrus fruits such as oranges and grape-fruit and rely instead on a choice of apples, grapes, pears, melon and occasionally a ripe banana.

Restoring bowel function

After the fast has been in operation for 24 hours or so the flow of chyme from the stomach into the small intestine will have ceased and so the bowel will be functioning less vigorously. Nevertheless, in a condition such as diverticulitis where the membranes are irritated and inflamed, the secretion of mucus may continue to be profuse for a time and there may be sporadic bouts of bowel looseness.

If, on the other hand, due to chronic constipation, bowel action continues to be sluggish some means must be employed to restore movement, either by resorting to the occasional use of an enema or by taking a herbal laxative. For the former purpose what is known as a gravity douche is likely to be the simplest and most effective apparatus for self-administration. This consists of a rubber bag, sometimes in the form of a hot-water bottle, fitted with a nozzle or adaptor to which one end of a rubber tube is connected. At the other end there is another nozzle and a tap or clip for controlling the flow of water. With the tap closed, the bag, containing a little more than ½ litre (1 pint) of warm water, is hung on the door of the toilet room at a height of 1½ metres (4 or 5 ft). The patient adopts a kneeling position with his or her back towards it. The nozzle, lubricated with a little soap or vegetable oil, is then inserted into the anus and, bending forward with his or her chest close to the floor, the patient releases the tap or clip and allows the water to flow into the rectum.

If the flow is too strong some griping or abdominal discomfort may be experienced, in which case the tap should be closed until the spasm eases. When the container is empty the patient should remain in the kneeling position for 2 or 3 minutes while kneading the abdomen gently with one hand. The nozzle is then removed and the bowel is emptied while continuing to massage the abdomen with the finger-tips, circling them in a clockwise direction up the right side, across just beneath the rib margins, down the left side, and back across to the right groin. Continue for several minutes until the bowel is emptied.

If there is difficulty in obtaining a gravity douche a bulb enema will serve as a suitable though slightly less convenient alternative. It consists of a length of tubing in the centre of which there is a rubber bulb which is squeezed to inject water from a bowl placed nearby on the floor.

One or other of these appliances should be obtainable from the surgical supplies department of the larger chemists' shops or from a surgical supplies store which can be located by reference to the local Yellow Pages telephone directory.

Should neither of these appliances be obtainable, however, a mild herbal laxative, available from health food stores, may be taken on rising for a day or two at the completion of the fast. Alternatively, a glass of one of the proprietary mineral waters, taken on rising and before retiring, may be found effective in some cases of moderate bowel sluggishness. Every effort should be made, however, to dispense with these artificial stimulants, and they should be resorted to only in cases of persistent constipation, otherwise there is a risk of becoming dependent on laxatives. As a consequence the bowel may be weakened by repeated purging and the restoration of a normal action could be impeded.

The latter can, however, be encouraged by two simple auxiliary procedures, the first of which, termed toilet drill, is explained in Appendix B on pages 110–112. The second is intended as a means of encouraging the adoption of a natural squatting position when using the toilet and so facilitating the operation of the muscular actions and nervous reflexes which combine to promote efficient bowel function. These anatomical prerequisites are partially or even totally obstructed by the upright sitting position which is necessitated by the design of the modern high-seated water closet which has only come into universal use during the past century or so. Prior to its introduction the act of defecation would have been performed by adopting a deep squatting position with the knees apart and the thighs flexed on the abdomen which is thus braced and supported to minimize strain when the muscles are contracted. At the same time the separation of the buttocks and the hollowing of the lumbar spine triggers off nervous reflexes which cause the anal sphincters to relax, while the muscular walls of the rectum are contracted so as to induce defecation.

In order to restore these conditions and counteract the inhibitory shortcomings of the standard toilet suite a compromise can be achieved by providing a platform to raise the feet between 7 and 10 cm (3 or 4 inches) and so flex the thighs on the abdomen. This can be achieved quite simply by placing two or three large books (e.g. telephone directories) just in front of the toilet pedestal. A more stable and permanent solution to the problem can take the form of a wooden platform such as the one illustrated in Figure 2. This can be made quite easily by anyone who has elementary carpentry facilities and skills. The measurements specified can be varied as necessary to meet personal requirements, but in practice it is likely that a platform height approximating to that mentioned previously will be found adequate.

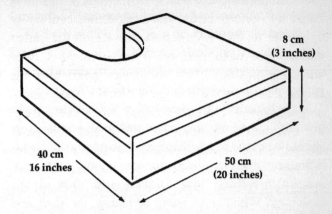

8 cm
(3 inches)

40 cm
16 inches

50 cm
(20 inches)

Figure 2 Toilet platform

Additional exercising

To further stimulate peristaltic action, counteract any distension of the abdominal muscles and stimulate pelvic circulation it is necessary in many cases to undertake a series of special remedial exercises. These are intended to supplement the regular daily walk or other outdoor activity which, as we have explained in a previous chapter, are a vital adjunct to an effective treatment programme. A sequence of suitable exercises is described and illustrated in Appendix A on pages 105–109 and these should be practised regularly and conscientiously at least once daily. Discretion should however be observed in the early stages of treatment to guard against the possibility of straining weakened muscles and supporting tissues. To this end the objective should be to keep well within the limitations of one's physical capacity, resting for a short time between movements and gradually extending the programme as strength and stamina are acquired.

If the benefits to be gained from the exercises are to be consolidated it is important that a conscious effort should be made to maintain good posture at all times. Slumping and stooping tend to cramp the chest, restrict breathing and weaken and distend the abdomen. Whether standing or sitting, the neck and spine should be kept as straight as possible and when walking the head should be held high and the abdominal muscles should be tightened. A comfortable, straight-backed chair should be preferred to a low, deep-cushioned armchair or settee.

Those who have observed our injunction to study carefully the anatomical and physiological principles outlined in earlier chapters will realize why we now stress the need to avoid any clothing or accessories which may cause constriction around the waist or thighs and so induce congestion in the lower limbs and abdomen by impeding the return circulation of blood and lymph. For this reason tight belts, suspenders and support garments and any garment which has a tight waistband should be dispensed with as far as possible in favour of clothing which is as light, loose-fitting and well-ventilated as circumstances and weather conditions permit.

Further remedial measures

To return to the subject of the treatment programme, there is another important remedial measure which needs to be introduced. It will be recalled that the healthy bowel is inhabited by beneficial bacteria, the function of which is not only to complete the digestion of proteins and carbohydrates but also to produce certain components of the vitamin B complex to supplement those extracted from our food. The colonies of these bacteria are often severely depleted when the bowel becomes inflamed and congested, and they may well have been totally destroyed if antibiotics have been taken in an effort to suppress existing symptoms or a previous illness. It is essential, therefore, that a healthy bacterial equilibrium should be restored as quickly as possible and this can be encouraged very effectively by including natural, unflavoured yogurt in the diet as soon as the fasting phase has been completed. Besides encouraging the regrowth and proliferation of the healthful bacteria this food has a mild laxative effect and also provides a small but readily digested amount of protein and calcium.

Another product which is useful in soothing inflamed mucous membranes and relieving flatulence is slippery elm food which is obtainable from health food stores and some chemists. Taken as a night-cap it promotes sound sleep and encourages peristalsis. It should be mixed to the consistency of a thin gruel with equal parts of skimmed milk and water and may be sweetened if desired with a teaspoon of honey.

It is not unusual during the early stages of treatment for some weight loss to occur, but this should not be a cause for concern since normal weight – as distinct from superfluous weight – will be restored as a result of the improvement in digestive and assimilative functions as the treatment progresses.

Guidelines for a dietary régime

The next objective, once the tissue-cleansing procedures have been completed, is to establish a dietary régime based on simple wholefoods which contain all the essential nutrients, in their natural proportions and combinations, as will be required to repair the damaged bowel tissues and restore their functional efficiency. This entails having a small, one-course meal consisting mainly of conservatively cooked vegetables, with an egg or cheese dish, which is eaten slowly and masticated thoroughly. This is supplemented with other small meals of raw or cooked fresh fruit or stewed or soaked dried fruit, and a little cereal food in the form of one or two slices of wholewheat bread or a dish of muesli (see recipe in Appendix C on page 118.

Both during treatment and subsequently it should be remembered that very hot foods and beverages can damage the mucous membranes of the alimentary canal and inhibit the secretion of gastric juices and enzymes. They should therefore be avoided, as also should household salt, pepper, vinegar and other condiments and sauces which impair digestive functions and have adverse effects on the nutrient properties of the foods. A little celery salt or yeast extract may be used for flavouring purposes if desired. A little honey may also be added to drinks, stewed fruits, etc., but sugar and synthetic sweeteners should not be used.

It is best for drinks to be taken between meals so as not to dilute the digestive juices, *but only sufficient to allay natural thirst.* It is a mistake to think that copious amounts of fluid should be taken 'to flush out the system'; they merely impose an unnecessary burden on the kidneys and bladder.

Fruit and vegetable juices, diluted with an equal quantity of water, are the most healthful and nutritious beverages. If possible they should be freshly prepared when needed with the aid of an electric juice extractor or a hand-operated juice-press, but unsweetened canned or bottled juices are a convenient and permissible alternative. They can be obtained from health food stores or some good chemists or general stores.

Meals which consist mainly of vegetables, fruits and wholegrain cereals are very nutritious and easily digested, but what is more important to the sufferer from diverticular disease is that they provide sufficient natural roughage to encourage the weakened intestine to resume peristaltic activity without undue strain.

Rest and relaxation

Bearing in mind what has been said in an earlier chapter concerning the damaging effects of mental stress on the body in general and the digestive system in particular, it will be appreciated why, at least during the early stages of treatment, care should be taken to rest and relax as much as possible. To this end, the aim should be to retire early, preferably in a darkened bedroom insulated as far as possible to exclude outside noise. Good ventilation is however essential to ensure that the air is not depleted of oxygen during sleep and so, if a window cannot be left ajar, the bedroom door should remain at least partially open.

A programme for treatment

In the next chapter all the components of the therapeutic régime outlined here will be incorporated into a progressive programme which can be followed on a day-by-day basis for a period of two weeks. Thereafter, the reader will be told how to consolidate any progress that has been made towards recovery, which will, of course, depend upon the extent of the damage which has been inflicted on the colon by diverticulitis in combination with other variables such as age, general health and any limitations imposed by domestic, occupational and other factors.

It would, of course, be unrealistic to expect speedy and dramatic improvements in a condition which has developed slowly over a period of many months – or even years. The initial aim is to cancel out the dietary and other obstructive factors which first led to a breakdown in the tissues of the colon and to establish an internal environment in which the body's self-healing and self-repairing powers can be mobilized and brought into effective action. Patience and perseverance will be called for, but, as has been stressed previously, any self-sacrifices which may be called for will surely be more than justified by the prospect of achieving a gradual improvement not only in respect of the bowel symptoms but of physical and systemic health generally.

From time to time it is to be expected that there will be what appear to be minor set-backs – the healing crises to which we referred previously and perhaps an occasional bout of abdominal discomfort or pain.

Should the latter occur, an effective means of obtaining relief is by the application of a hot compress. For this purpose a piece of cotton material, old sheeting, for example, is folded into four or five thicknesses, wrung out in hot water and applied to the abdomen and covered with a dry towel to retain the heat. When circumstances permit, it is best to retire to bed with a hot-water bottle at the feet. The compress should be reheated from time to time, but if necessary it can remain in place throughout the night. The compress material should be rinsed thoroughly after use.

Although heat is useful for the relief of local pain, it is unwise to indulge in frequent hot baths because they tend to weaken the blood vessels, cause circulatory congestion and increase susceptibility to chilling. A moderately hot bath may be taken once weekly, but in order to tone up the blood vessels and stimulate the circulation a cool or cold sponge-down should be taken each morning, followed by a brisk friction-rub with a loofah, or coarse towel, or a skin-brush. The sponge-down and friction-rub should also be taken after the weekly hot bath. The initial shock caused by the cold application is very quickly replaced by a glowing, warm reaction which is reinforced by the physical activity of the friction-rub.

Where the symptoms of diverticulitis are of recent origin, i.e. in those who suffer only occasional bouts of abdominal discomfort, constipation and diarrhoea, it is reasonable to expect that there will be progressive improvement in the course of a few months. In long-standing and more severe cases, however, the whole course of treatment will almost certainly have to be repeated at intervals of two or three months before normal bowel functions are restored.

8
Now let's get started

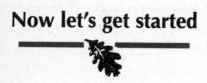

I t is now time to summarize the various treatment
measures which have been explained in the preceding chapters and set out a daily programme
covering a period of two weeks or so. During this
time the initial short fast will have cleared the bowel
of any overload of food residues, and the alkalizing
diet will have soothed the inflamed mucous membranes and helped to restore a more efficient peristaltic action.

What we are proposing should *not,* however, be
regarded as a once-and-for-all 'cure'. For, as we hope
the reader will by now have fully appreciated, if health
is to be maintained and a recurrence of the bowel
problems is to be prevented, it is imperative that what
has been achieved shall be consolidated and sustained
by avoiding a recession into the harmful habits and

practices which were responsible for the original breakdown.

Consequently, at the conclusion of the active treatment programme a balanced, wholefood dietary régime needs to be adopted, based on the specimen menus set out in Appendix C on pages 113–119. Equally every effort should be made to maintain good muscle tone and circulatory efficiency by continuing to take as much outdoor exercise as possible and minimizing mental and physical stress as far as is practicable.

If during the initial two weeks of the programme domestic or occupational commitments necessitate some adjustments to the time-sequence in which the therapeutic measures are set out, minor variations may be made provided that the dietary instructions are complied with conscientiously. It is permissible, for example, to transpose meals but *not* to alter their components, and the exercise sessions may be incorporated into the daily routine at whatever times are most convenient.

Once again, however, we would urge that any doubts concerning the nature and purpose of any of the treatment measures should be thoroughly dispelled by reading and rereading the appropriate preceding chapters. With that final injunction we can now embark on the road to recovery.

Daily treatment programme

1st day

1 *On rising*: Toilet drill (see Appendix B, pages 110–112).
2 Glass of water or diluted juice, sipped slowly. No solid food or other liquids *of any kind* may be taken throughout the day.
3 Have a cool or cold sponge-down followed by friction-rub.
4 Carry out abdominal exercises detailed in Appendix A, pages 103–107.
5 Take outdoor exercise if possible, such as a half-hour walk combined with deep breathing. On return, have sponge-down and friction-rub and change clothing if necessary.
6 Glass of water or juice if thirsty.
7 Rest for half hour or more if possible.
8 Carry on with necessary activities during the day, but try to avoid any which involve undue mental or physical strain. Rest occasionally, if possible, preferably in a darkened room.
9 *Early evening:* Take outdoor exercise if possible.
10 *Before retiring:* Carry out remedial exercises and toilet drill, followed by moderately hot bath if desired to promote relaxation, and retire early.

2nd and 3rd days

Repeat the first-day schedule but if tiredness or 'healing crisis' symptoms are experienced omit outdoor exercise and sponge-down and rest as much as possible. Use the enema or take a herbal laxative on the third day if there has not been a natural bowel movement.

4th day

1 *On rising*: Carry out toilet drill.
2 Drink of water or diluted juice.
3 Have sponge-down and friction-rub.
4 Carry out abdominal exercises.
5 *Breakfast:* Five or six stewed prunes or some stewed apple with 140 ml (¼ pint) of unflavoured yogurt.
6 Take outdoor exercise if desired, and sponge-down and friction-rub.
7 Drinks as needed between meals.
8 *Midday:* Same as breakfast or an apple, a pear and a few grapes if preferred (remove the pips from the latter).
9 Carry out any necessary normal activities, but rest when possible.
10 *Early evening:* Repeat midday meal, and take outdoor exercise if desired followed by sponge-down and friction-rub.

11 *Before retiring:* Abdominal exercises followed by moderately hot bath if desired. Toilet drill, and enema if necessary. A cup of slippery elm food.

5th and 6th days

Repeat the fourth day's schedule, but outdoor exercise should be taken at least once during the day. If still constipated use the enema or laxative provided that has not been needed on either day three or four.

7th and 8th days

The following programme should be adapted to fit in with ordinary domestic or other commitments.

1 *On rising:* Glass of water or juice, toilet drill, abdominal exercises, sponge-down and friction-rub.
2 *Breakfast:* Fruit and yogurt as on previous days.
3 Outdoor exercise if possible; sponge-down and friction-rub.
4 *Midday:* Fruit and yogurt as on previous days, but a ripe banana should replace one of the other items.
5 Outdoor exercise, sponge-down and friction-rub.
6 *Evening meal:* Small serving of two or three conservatively cooked root or green vegetables, e.g. cabbage, sprouts, carrots, parsnips, onion, but *not*

potatoes, with a tablespoon of cottage cheese or a scrambled or lightly poached egg.

7 *Before retiring*: Abdominal exercises; toilet drill. A cup of slippery elm food.

9th and 10th days

Continue as on preceding days except:
Evening meal: Have a conservatively cooked or baked jacket potato together with two other vegetables and a poached or scrambled egg, or a small omelette, or one tablespoon of cream cheese.

An enema or laxative should be used only if there has been no bowel movement during the previous 48 hours.

11th to 14th days

Continue as before except:

1 *Midday meal:* Have a small mixed salad of lettuce, tomato, watercress, grated raw carrot, etc., 30 g (1 oz) washed sultanas or raisins, sprinkled with 60 g (2 oz) grated cheese or 30 g (1 oz) grated nuts (e.g. almonds, walnuts, hazelnuts, peanuts, etc.). Remember to eat slowly and masticate thoroughly, but if any digestive discomfort should be experienced revert to fruit and yogurt the following day.

2 The weekly hot bath may be taken before retiring or in the morning if preferred, in which case it should be followed by the sponge-down and friction-rub.

3 It should be possible by now to dispense with the enema, but the herbal laxative or mineral water may be resorted to every four or five days until a regular bowel action is re-established.

15th day

1 *On rising:* Glass of water or juice, toilet drill, abdominal exercises and sponge-down and friction-rub.

2 *Breakfast:* Choose from menus in Appendix C on pages 113–119.

3 Continue to take drinks of water or juice as needed between meals, but a cup or two of weak, unsweetened tea or decaffeinated coffee may be taken instead during the day.

4 *Midday:* Choose from menus in Appendix C.

5 Take outdoor exercise at any convenient time, aiming to extend its duration to a total of one hour whenever possible. Have sponge-down and friction-rub on return.

6 *Evening meal:* Choose from menus in Appendix C.

7 *Before retiring:* Abdominal exercises. Cup of slippery elm food if desired.

9

Consolidate!

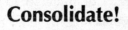

Diverticular disease, as we have stressed repeatedly, is not something that has been 'caught' but is the result of long-continued dietetic and other errors as a result of which the complex chemistry of the various parts of the alimentary canal has been disrupted and the tissues of the bowel have been weakened and finally eroded.

It has to be recognized, therefore, that time and patience will be needed to repair damaged tissues and restore metabolic balance. In the end, however, it is only through the reader's understanding of the nature of his or her problems and determination to achieve a lasting solution that eventual salvation will come. An added bonus is the realization that the reward for a relatively short-term sacrifice and some changes in established habits and routines is not merely relief from distressing bowel symptoms but the restoration of the body's very efficient defence mechanisms which, when they are functioning effectively, will ensure a high degree of immunity from other organic and systemic disorders.

The specimen menus which are set out in Appendix C are, of course, intended to exemplify the type of meals which will adequately meet the nutritional needs of many readers, but provided that the basic 60:20:20 ratio is observed, (as explained on page 72), there is scope for considerable variation in the choice of main dishes. Remember, however, to choose *whole*, unprocessed and natural foods whenever possible, not to over-eat, not to have a large meal if tired or under stress, and to eat slowly and masticate thoroughly.

Finally, if further help is needed in choosing recipes and arranging healthy meals, a catalogue of excellent wholefood cookery books is available from the publishers and a selection of these will usually be found on the shelves of health food stores and good bookshops.

Appendix A

Abdominal Exercises

These exercises are designed to strengthen the muscles of the abdomen and reduce distension. For the maximum benefit they should be practised twice daily – on rising and during the evening, but not less than one hour after a meal.

If at first any movement proves to be beyond one's physical capacity it should be omitted from the programme for a time, concentrating instead on the less demanding movements.

The aim should be to *develop the muscles progressively* by gradually increasing the range of movement and the number of repetitions, taking care to avoid undue strain. Initially, one or two repetitions of each movement may be all that can be achieved, but over a period of several weeks it should be possible to manage between ten and twenty repetitions, depending upon the nature of the exercise and the patient's innate physical resources.

1 Lie on the back with the hands resting on the lower abdomen and raise the legs slowly, keeping the knees straight, until the feet are clear of the floor, then lower and relax. The abdominal muscles will be felt to contract and harden as the legs are raised and then relax and soften when they are lowered. As the abdomen becomes stronger, the legs can be held in the raised position for a few seconds before returning to the starting position.

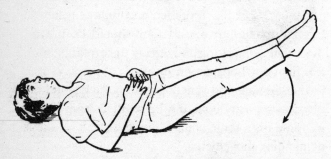

2 From the same starting position but with the arms splayed and the hands pressing on the floor, raise the legs to the vertical position with the knees straight, then separate them as widely as possible and close again, pressing the knees and ankles together strongly, repeating three or four times before lowering the legs and relaxing.

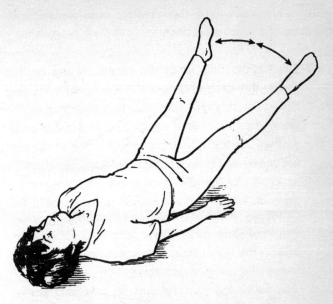

3 Lie on the back with the feet anchored and the hands resting on the lower abdomen, then rise slowly to a sitting position, return to starting position and relax.

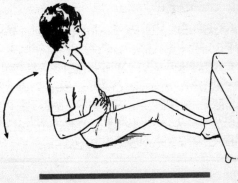

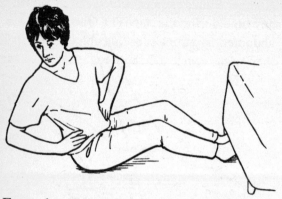

4 From the same starting position, raise the head and shoulders clear of the floor and rotate them first to the right, then to the left, and then return to starting position and relax.

5 The following exercise can be practised conveniently and unobtrusively at any time when seated in a comfortable high-backed chair or settee and it serves as a useful auxiliary means of consolidating the benefits of the main exercise programme. Settle comfortably with the head and shoulders resting against the back of the chair, place the hands with the fingers pressing gently into the lower abdomen, then simply move the head and shoulders forward two or three inches, hold for a few seconds, then return to the starting position and relax. The abdominal muscles will be felt to contract and relax alternately.

6 Another simple exercise which can be practised at any time during the day is as follows: draw in the abdomen as strongly as possible while inhaling, then release while exhaling. Repeat as convenient.

Appendix B
Toilet drill

Following defecation the rectum normally remains empty until such time as the terminal part of the colon is refilled and the need for the bowel to be emptied is signalled once again. When, in response to this signal, the natural squatting position is adopted, nerve reflexes initiate peristaltic contractions in the colon which propel the faeces into the rectum. The distension created by this triggers another nerve reflex which causes the anal sphincters to relax and so permit the free passage of the faeces which the rectal muscles are voluntarily contracted.

In order to stimulate these reflexes when the bowel has become sluggish, a simple 'toilet drill' should be carried out as follows:

When seated on the toilet with the feet raised (as advised on page 86), the body should be bent forward so that the thighs compress and support the abdomen and then the hands are placed behind the back with the finger-tips touching just above the anus. Then, pressing gently but firmly, the fingers are pulled upwards and outwards, so as to accentuate the spread of the buttocks, while at the same time contracting and pressing down with the abdominal muscles for 3 or 4 seconds. Relax the hand-pressure and abdominal muscles for a few more seconds, then repeat the sequence rhythmically, continuing for up to 10 minutes or until a bowel movement is achieved.

The drill should be practised twice daily, on rising and just before retiring, with the object of establishing a regular bowel rhythm.

In cases of chronic constipation the faeces may have become hard and impacted in the distended colon and so prevented from entering the rectum and triggering the nerve reflexes which initiate peristalsis and relax the anal sphincters. This problem may sometimes be resolved by means of the following technique:

A piece of thin but strong plastic, approximately 12 cm (15 inches) square (the corner cut from a plastic bag is better) is placed over the forefinger which, after being lubricated with a little soap or vegetable oil, is inserted gently 2 or 3 cm (an inch or so) into the anus and slowly circled around exerting firm pressure on the mucous membranes just inside the empty rectum.

Rhythmic contraction of the abdominal muscles will help to move the impacted faeces into the rectum and the finger can then be withdrawn.

Appendix C

A week's menus

The following menus are intended to exemplify the type of balanced wholefood meals which will satisfy most 'normal' appetites and meet all the body's nutritional needs. Some adjustments are permissible, however, in regard to the protein components of the main meals and the size of the servings in relation to such variables as physical characteristics, age, and work-loads imposed by occupational, recreational and sporting activities.

Non-vegetarians may substitute 80 or 90 g (3 oz) of meat, fish or poultry for the protein element of the meal, but care should be taken to avoid over-eating and to ensure that the overall 60:20:20 ratios are maintained.

Any fruits, vegetables or salads which are not in season may be replaced by similar items. Fruit should always be fully ripe; sour or unripe produce should *never* be eaten either raw or cooked.

Commercial 'salad creams,' dressings, sauces, table salt and other condiments should never be used, although a little celery salt – obtainable from health food stores – may be added during cooking if desired, as also may yeast extract. Salads may be dressed with a little yogurt or a dessertspoonful of vegetable oil mixed with a teaspoon of fresh lemon or orange juice.

If at first wholewheat bread tends to cause indigestion or flatulence, a lower-extraction loaf may be substituted, i.e. one of those described as 'brown', 'granary', 'farmhouse', etc. Revert gradually to 100 per cent wholewheat bread as digestive tolerance is improved.

1st day

Breakfast   Stewed prunes or other dried fruit sprinkled with a dessertspoonful of wheat-germ and served with 140 ml (¼ pint) unflavoured yogurt.

Midday   Three slices of wholewheat bread spread with mashed ripe banana and washed sultanas or raisins; an apple of pear or a few grapes.

Evening   Mixed salad (see recipe on page 117).

2nd day

Breakfast Muesli (see recipe on page 118).

Midday Lettuce and chopped celery with cottage cheese, sprinkled with washed raisins or sultanas.

Evening Millet savoury (see recipe on page 118) with steamed cabbage and carrots.

3rd day

Breakfast Fresh fruit, e.g. two or three items chosen from apples, oranges, pears, grapes or oranges.

Midday Two slices of wholewheat toast or crisp-bread with cottage cheese or peanut butter, or yeast extract, and an apple or pear.

Evening Plain omelette with two steamed green or root vegetables.

4th day

Breakfast Half grapefruit sweetened if necessary with a little melted honey, and 140 ml (¼ pint) natural yogurt and sliced banana.

Midday Scrambled egg on wholewheat toast.

Evening Mixed vegetable casserole sprinkled with 50 g (2 oz) grated cheese.

5th day

Breakfast Muesli
Midday Stewed apple with chopped dates or raisins and yogurt.
Evening Cauliflower cheese with two medium potatoes and carrots or peas.

6th day

Breakfast Poached or scrambled egg with two slices of wholewheat toast.
Midday Small salad, e.g. lettuce, grated carrot, tomato and 30 g (1 oz) washed raisins or sultanas.
Evening Two nut cutlets (mixture obtainable from health food stores) with steamed carrots and spinach or other green vegetable.

7th day

Breakfast Fruit salad, e.g. sliced ripe banana, chopped apple or pear, washed raisins or sultanas or chopped dates, with 140 ml (¼ pint) yogurt.
Midday Two slices of crispbread or wholewheat toast, spread thinly with yeast extract, and 60 g (2 oz) cheese and an apple, pear or orange.
Evening Mixed salad (see recipe below)

Recipes

Mixed Salad

Lettuce leaves, washed
Tomato, sliced
Carrot, grated
Cucumber, sliced
Celery, chopped
Beetroot (raw or cooked – no vinegar), grated or
  sliced
Watercress
½ medium apple
1 dessertspoon washed dried fruit (sultanas, raisins,
  chopped dates, etc.)
50 g (2 oz) cheese
50 g (2 oz) nuts (peanuts, almonds, hazelnuts, etc.)
½ ripe banana, sliced.

1 Tear the lettuce leaves into pieces and use to line a
  large plate.
2 Decorate with the tomato, carrot, cucumber, celery, beetroot and watercress – you can use whatever selection of salads are available.
3 Dice the apple finely and scatter over, together
  with the dried fruit.
4 Grate the cheese and nuts and sprinkle over, then
  decorate with the banana slices.

Muesli

1 heaped dessertspoon washed raisins, sultanas of chopped dates
2 or 3 heaped dessertspoons coarse oatmeal
1 level dessertspoon honey (optional)
4 dessertspoons warm water or half skimmed milk and water
½ medium apple, finely chopped
2 heaped dessertspoons grated nuts (peanuts, almonds, hazelnuts, etc.)
½ ripe banana, sliced

1 Mix the dried fruit into the oatmeal.
2 Melt the honey (if used) in the warm water and pour over the oatmeal. Leave to soak for 1 hour or overnight.
3 Before serving add the apple, sprinkle over the nuts and decorate with the banana slices.

Millet Savoury

3 medium tomatoes, skinned and sliced
1 clove garlic, crushed (optional)
275 ml (½ pint) water
1 level teaspoon yeast extract
2 tablespoons millet
Chopped parsley

1 Put the tomatoes, skinned and sliced, in a pan with the crushed garlic. Pour over the water, stir in the yeast extract and bring to the boil.
2 Add the millet, stir well, then cover and simmer until the water is absorbed – approximately 15 minutes.
3 Just before serving, sprinkle with the chopped parsley.

Index